Patients Making Meaning

I0050672

This book explores how women make meaning at various health flashpoints in their lives, overcoming fear, anxiety, and anger to draw upon self-advocacy, research, and crucial decision-making.

Combining focus group research, content analysis, autoethnography, and textual inquiry, the book argues that the making and remaking of what we call "patient epistemologies" is a continual process wherein a health flashpoint—sometimes a new diagnosis, sometimes a reoccurrence or worsening of an existing condition or the progression of a natural process—can cause an individual to be thrust into a discourse community that was not of their own choosing.

This study will interest students and scholars of health communication, rhetoric of health and medicine, women's studies, public health, healthcare policy, philosophy of medicine, medical sociology, and medical humanities.

Bryna Siegel Finer is Professor of English at Indiana University of Pennsylvania, USA, where she serves as the Director of Undergraduate Writing Programs. She is the co-editor of *Writing Program Architecture* and *Women's Health Advocacy*.

Cathryn Molloy is Professor of Writing Studies in the English department at the University of Delaware, USA. She is the author of *Rhetorical Ethos in Health and Medicine: Patient Credibility, Stigma, and Misdiagnosis* and is co-editor of the *Rhetoric of Health and Medicine* journal.

Jamie White-Farnham is Professor in the Writing Program at University of Wisconsin-Superior, USA, where she serves as Director of Teaching & Learning. She is the co-editor of *Writing Program Architecture* and *Women's Health Advocacy*.

Routledge Studies in Rhetoric and Communication

Patients Making Meaning

Theorizing Sources of Information and Forms of Support in Women's Health

Bryna Siegel Finer, Cathryn Molloy, and Jamie White-Farnham

Routledge
Taylor & Francis Group

NEW YORK AND LONDON

First published 2024
by Routledge
605 Third Avenue, New York, NY 10158

and by Routledge
4 Park Square, Milton Park, Abingdon, Oxon OX14 4RN

Routledge is an imprint of the Taylor & Francis Group, an informa business

© 2024 Bryna Siegel Finer, Cathryn Molloy, and Jamie White-Farnham

The right of Bryna Siegel Finer, Cathryn Molloy, and Jamie White-Farnham to be identified as authors of this work has been asserted in accordance with sections 77 and 78 of the Copyright, Designs and Patents Act 1988.

All rights reserved. No part of this book may be reprinted or reproduced or utilised in any form or by any electronic, mechanical, or other means, now known or hereafter invented, including photocopying and recording, or in any information storage or retrieval system, without permission in writing from the publishers.

Trademark notice: Product or corporate names may be trademarks or registered trademarks, and are used only for identification and explanation without intent to infringe.

Library of Congress Cataloging-in-Publication Data
Names: Finer, Bryna Siegel, author. | Molloy, Cathryn, author. | White-Farnham, Jamie, author.
Title: Patients making meaning : theorizing sources of information and forms of support in women's health / by Bryna Siegel Finer, Cathryn Molloy, Jamie White-Farnham.
Description: New York, NY : Routledge, 2024. | Series: Routledge studies in rhetoric and communication | Includes bibliographical references and index.
Identifiers: LCCN 2023032239 (print) | LCCN 2023032240 (ebook) | ISBN 9781032503943 (hardback) | ISBN 9781032503967 (paperback) | ISBN 9781003398318 (ebook)
Subjects: LCSH: Women--Health and hygiene--Social aspects. | Communication in medicine. | Women--Health and hygiene--Information services. | Women patients--Social conditions--21st century. | Women's health services--Social aspects.
Classification: LCC RA564.85 .F557 2024 (print) | LCC RA564.85 (ebook) | DDC 610.1/4--dc23/eng/20230719
LC record available at https://lccn.loc.gov/2023032239
LC ebook record available at https://lccn.loc.gov/2023032240

ISBN: 978-1-032-50394-3 (hbk)
ISBN: 978-1-032-50396-7 (pbk)
ISBN: 978-1-003-39831-8 (ebk)

DOI: 10.4324/9781003398318

Typeset in Times New Roman
by Deanta Global Publishing Services, Chennai, India

We dedicate this book to Nedra Reynolds, who taught us in and beyond the classroom to be thoughtful writers, readers, teachers, and scholars in rhetoric and composition. We are better because of your guidance and support.

Contents

Illustrations

Acknowledgments

We decided to write a book on women's health rhetoric in Fall 2019. Nothing could have prepared us for the simultaneous gut punch of the global health crisis and a second cancer diagnosis for Bryna during early 2020. Amid the challenges of keeping safe and healthy, schooling for our children (that year ages 2–18), our own and our spouses' professional and work lives being upended (including in universities, K–12 education, and healthcare contexts), and all our own, our spouses', our students, and our own children's mental health, our inquiry seemed more relevant than ever: what do people need during a health flashpoint?

The book came together slowly but surely, a feat we chalk up to friendship and the unique and inspiring thrill that the study of people's stories, language, and rhetoric brings. We know this is true because between June and December 2020, over 50 women contributed to this project as research participants with us. Our gratitude to them is immeasurable.

We thank Zoom. We hate Zoom, but it was instrumental to our connection, conversation, and focus during those hard times.

We thank our research assistant, Adrianna Ladd, whose careful eye made this book stronger. We also thank Ruby Farnham for her graphic design support.

We thank our supportive colleagues at James Madison University, Indiana University of Pennsylvania, and the University of Wisconsin-Superior, as well as Rhetoric of Health and Medicine (RHM) mentors Lisa Melançon, J. Blake Scott, and Fred Reynolds, and our mentors from the University of Rhode Island.

We thank the team at Routledge, especially Suzanne Richardson and Stuti Goel.

We thank our families including our husbands Steve Farnham, David Finer, and Jimmy Raisch, as well as our children Lucas and Mateo Raisch, Ruby and Claire Farnham, and Theo Finer.

We thank each other. There is something special about being women, friends, rhetoricians, rhetoricians of health and medicine, writers, and all those things together at the same time. Working together continues to challenge us, teach us new things, push our imaginations, and write, the thing we all love the most. We are grateful that our professional paths are aligned and intertwined and that we work in conditions that allow us to collaborate across three states and two time zones, amid and because of global strife.

We greatly appreciate the opportunity to write this book. It helped us stick together as we worked through health challenges to articulate important personal stuff that we think will help other people through the lens of rhetoric, which brought us together in the first place.

1 Starting from friendship and rhetoric

An introduction to patient epistemology

We start with Restaino (2019), who writes,

> I ask here that, as researchers and writers, we find greater analytical
> space for love, for friendship, for care, for being changed and lost and
> rewritten ourselves in the research process.... Friendship and love are,
> too, fertile ground for the study of rhetoric.
>
> (p. 25)

Friendship and care begin this story and book. Our friendship began alongside our study of rhetoric a few days before the beginning of the semester in
2004, when Bryna walked through the double doors of Roosevelt Hall on
the campus of the University of Rhode Island to find Cathryn sitting on a
flower-upholstered sofa searching through her backpack; their friendship was
instantaneous. Two years later, as tutors in the university writing center in the
same stuffy building, we met Jamie. In all, the three of us have been friends
for twenty years, through weddings, babies, multiple job changes, kids head-
ing off into the world; we've presented together at conferences, co-authored
articles, co-edited books, and supported each other during individual health
crises and the global pandemic.

Health crises are unfortunately central in our friendship and in our work as
rhetoricians of health and medicine. Our personal and academic conversations
surrounding health are mainly centered on Bryna's health because in 2005,
she was found to be a carrier of the BRCA2 gene mutation, and in 2013 she
was diagnosed with ductal carcinoma in situ, precancerous cells in the milk
ducts in her right breast. She underwent a mastectomy and reconstruction,
which necessitated several months of recovery and resulted in years of discomfort and related health problems. She was diagnosed with stage IIa breast
cancer in her reconstructed right breast six years later at the age of forty-three.
This shocking news came in the early days of the pandemic when we were
isolated, recovering from the "online pivot" of spring 2020 for all our kids
(then in pre-school, elementary, high school, and freshman year of college),
and of course our own universities' pivots and fall planning. Bryna spent that

DOI: 10.4324/9781003398318-1

fall semester recovering from surgery and going through chemotherapy. She spent most of the spring 2020 semester in daily radiation treatments. Throughout this time, Cathryn and Jamie of course listened and supported Bryna through many emotions and physical challenges of undergoing breast cancer treatment during the pandemic. Being rhetoricians, our conversations often tended to also include appraisals and analyses of the many discourses that surrounded Bryna as a patient, such as the dogmatic medical documents given to her at the hospital and the support group packages sent or delivered to her that included things like flyers and glossy magazines. Bryna began to collect this ephemera in a binder, then a whole drawer.

In addition, friends and family reached out in various ways, whether through email, texts, cards in the mail, or phone calls. Unsurprisingly, many cards and messages would include the ever-present pink ribbon, which grated on all our nerves. Surprisingly, some of these messages and offers of support were odd or not exactly what Bryna had in mind in terms of help. When she needed someone to babysit her son, Theo, so she could attend appointments, relatives were eager to send her jewelry and other gifts as a treat to herself. In order to keep friends and family in the loop on the progress of her treatment as well as be honest about what she needed and what was not helpful to her, Bryna created a Facebook group with the banner "Fuck Cancer." In this space with an audience of people she could be honest with, Bryna could share information and gain support that did not smack of warrior clichés.

Over the duration of Bryna's treatment, our casual analyses of various patient support materials and well-wisher messages grew in coherence and began to crystallize into lines of inquiry. Rather than just critiquing, we were interested in learning what types of messages and materials actually would help patients understand, feel supported, and make meaning during and from their health and medical experiences—we wished to understand these things and, in doing so, eventually theorized a *patient epistemology*, or the actions taken throughout a health journey through which people make meaning: perceiving, reading, watching, listening, asking questions, talking, learning, weighing evidence, making decisions, complaining, expressing gratitude, expressing doubt, and critiquing—among other discursive modes and acts.

Of course, for many years, research has been published on patient education materials (PEM), which look at how patients understand documents meant to inform them about their illnesses. These studies have primarily looked at usability and reading-level (see, for two examples, Öresland et al., 2015; Lipari et al., 2019). Additionally, there are many publications in the field of the rhetoric of health and medicine (RHM) and in the popular reading market devoted to patient narratives, especially around breast cancer. These are valuable for the centering of women's voices and for the way they can inspire other patients, but they can suffer from—as critics such as Judy Z. Segal have demonstrated, and chapters in this book will also reflect—stagnation and even agnotology, the cultural production of ignorance (Segal, 2008).

Therefore, we considered much more than just one type of discourse, such as narratives, in regard to and aimed at patients within *rhetorical encounters*, or the instances in which women consume and/or are confronted with a huge variety of texts, messages, patient education materials, informative videos on YouTube, cancer blogs and social media accounts, plus messages of all types from friends, family, co-workers, and other patients in online support spaces. These encounters are part of and often spark certain emotional, affective, constitutive, and meaning-making effects, whether intentionally sought by the patient or not, whether helpful or not. From experience, we know that when facing a certain medical situation, whether an acute disease or a chronic condition, patients can be overwhelmed by the high number of messages and materials they receive from doctors, social workers, support groups, and loved ones. These materials, while intended to inform, help, and support the patient, can have a variety of *epistemological consequences*: the results of rhetorical knowledge-making often unintended by the author/creator of the document.

Epistemological consequences are more than a simple understanding of literal words and phrases. An interaction with a certain message can constitute a rhetorical encounter that significantly affects the patient's worldview or identity: an epistemological consequence. Because epistemology is discursive and rhetorical in nature and occurs within interactions of ideas, language, information, and symbols, rhetorical encounters set a scene for meaning-making. The experience of encountering, reacting to, and potentially engaging in a health discourse at a time when one is inducted into it because of a health flashpoint, such as being diagnosed with a life-threatening disease, can be less purposeful or within a person's control than we might expect or want to believe is so as feminists. Such presumptions are informed by dominant discourses that have their ways of permeating the culture and hence shaping beliefs and understandings that are hard to avoid.

As one case from our study demonstrates, for instance, choosing reconstruction after mastectomy is not presented by the medical establishment as a true choice in the moment despite other options. Had the messages and materials not perpetuated the norm of reconstructed breasts, at least one of our participants in our study would have chosen "flat closure" after her surgery, as the aesthetics of a flat chest would have aligned better with her gender identity. She could only know this after reflecting on her experience, imbued as it was with worry, a hurried pace, and limited knowledge of the wider conversation around mastectomy closure choices within the rhetorical encounters she by chance experienced.

This book is thusly catalyzed by our shared attention to rhetorical and epistemological questions during the lived experiences of Bryna's cancer diagnoses and treatments, as well as Jamie and Cathryn's lived experiences in other health realms, all of us as both audience members of many health messages and materials and feminist researchers wishing to learn: what *are* the best ways to support people, what *are* the appropriate messages, and what *do* women want when they are suffering through a painful and scary health flashpoint? Our interest in theorizing a patient epistemology by studying rhetorical encounters and their epistemological consequences during a health flashpoint began with these research questions:

- what discourses do women encounter and from whom during health flashpoints, meaning mainly acute or onset health diagnoses, which sometimes set off a personal crisis?
- how do women interact with these materials and messages?
- what sorts of materials and messages help women make meaning during an illness or health crisis?
- what sorts of materials and messages hinder them if any?
- what does any meaning-making bring to bear on the women's decisions, relationships, identities, and understandings of their health?

To address these questions, we undertook a study utilizing several research methodologies that innervate the RHM with attention to four main bodies of evidence: survey and focus groups of women who have had breast cancer; textual analyses of two different health discourses surrounding women, and our lived experiences, all of which will be explained presently. From our inquiry, we have learned that meaning-making is an iterative process that begins with rhetorical encounters with a variety of discourses (PEM, cultural narratives, well-wishes, etc.). The initial encounter is followed by an affective response which influences rhetorical work (such as reading, talking, listening, decision-making, emoting, etc.), and which creates effects on both a local, personal level as well as a global, societal level. Both actions shape and project epistemological frameworks, which can alternately inspire, limit, help, and hurt. Over time and as a person's health status changes, improves, worsens, etc., understandings and identities continue to change upon reflection. In fact, this process probably does not end in a person's life in regard to how health discourses will resonate after a life-changing health flashpoint.

The description of this process is our main finding and claim of this book. Each chapter illustrates the terms we have introduced here and provides examples of how rhetorical encounters have shaped patients' epistemologies and material lives in various health situations. The difficulty of that type of rhetorical work within this process is demonstrable across several examples of women's health concerns, both on personal and social levels. Our data and examples illustrate the variety of discourses, the clarity and also confusion of available epistemological frameworks, and their effects on the understandings, actions, identities, and rhetorical choices of women who have undergone breast cancer treatment, experienced menopause, and sought sobriety.

Staking out the ground: from discourse community to rhetorical community

The concept of a discourse community has been an important one, both explicitly and implicitly, in RHM literature; in some writings, "discourse community" is invoked in terms of the academic discourse community (Melonçon & Scott, 2018; Reed, 2018; Reynolds, 2018). In other work, even when the phrase "discourse community" is rarely or never explicitly used, the idea of a discourse community that patients enter into (sometimes unwittingly) is implied (Kessler, 2022; Pender, 2018). In undertaking our study, we were initially drawn to the idea of "discourse community" since, undoubtedly, women enter into new discourse communities of various kinds when they receive any of a myriad of diagnoses and then make their way through treatments and aftercare. We know discourse communities are comprised of people who connect rhetorically—through specialized vocabulary, jokes, tropes, ways of sharing, and expectations for contributing to and benefitting from the community. However, the term is limited in its capacity to help us conceptualize and communicate the emotional and affective dimensions of some health and medical situations that are highly personal and individual and at the same time, communal and shared in nature.

While the term "discourse community" comes close to explaining how, for instance, breast cancer patients share their experiences, especially in online support spaces, it is not a perfect fit here since we are looking at patients' experiences encountering a variety of types of messages and materials aimed at them, and we are not looking at the actual medical stories and experiences of the patients themselves. In fact, we called on our participants to join us as rhetorical analysts in order for them to tell us what messages and materials evinced certain reactions, emotions, and (mis)understandings.

To better capture how meaning is made from these patients' (and our own) experiences as women in health and medical situations, we draw on the ancient rhetorical concept of *nomos*—a term whose history and feminist reclamation we discuss presently. We use *nomos* to refer to communal meaning-making born of personal experience with and between the poles of logos and mythos. Connecting "nomos" to "discourse community" allowed us to develop a new coinage, a *rhetorical community*.

Rhetorical communities are groups of people inducted into a realm of discourse which they may or may not participate in as rhetors themselves. More than simply an audience, however, rhetorical community members are both the expressed consumers of and profoundly in need of the discourse (such as medical information). The stakes of membership are quite high, as we have begun to suggest, as there are epistemological consequences of the rhetorical encounters in the rhetorical community. Rhetorical communities are also unlike a discourse community in two key ways: most often, induction into a discourse community is predicated on the person's ability and willingness (or hope or plan) to participate in the rhetorical rules and ways of discoursing in the community (such as a scholarly discipline or fandom). However, there is no such choice or desire for participation in a rhetorical community, since induction often comes amid life-altering, shatteringly bad news; these are some of the worst moments of someone's life, and so induction into this rhetorical community is unwanted or perhaps even resisted.

In some ways, what we are attempting to express resembles Molly Kessler's (2022) *Stigma Stories: Rhetoric, Lived Experience, and Chronic Illness* in which she convincingly argues that stigma—at times visceral, nearly always steeped in affect—is as much a part of living with a chronic condition as the condition itself; one cannot be disentangled from the other. In the same way, we track the affect that is always a part of a health flashpoint and is neither separate nor separable from the rhetorical work that needs to happen following a new diagnosis, a flare of an existing condition, or a new life phase. Just as Kessler's work helps those in RHM to consider how stigma operates on a number of levels such that ways to work against stigma open up, our project examines the process of patient epistemologies such that ways to purposefully and impactfully intervene in that process can open up. Like Kessler's work, our work in this book is better served by the idea of a rhetorical community rather than a discourse community as in neither case is there a choice to opt in; induction is thrust upon a person.

Thus, we offer our participants who have been diagnosed and treated for breast cancer as an example of a rhetorical community. Upon diagnosis, they are inducted into the community (and there may be several, for instance, depending on the type(s) of breast cancer, type(s) of treatment, etc.) at first as audience members at which so many messages, materials, and resources from the medical, public, and philanthropic spheres are aimed. There is a range of reactions to these messages; some patients embrace certain discourses and incorporate them into their meaning-making and identities. They become previvors or eventually survivors, and their friends and families become prayer warriors. Others are angered by the "pink-washing" of the breast cancer support industrial complex, rejecting the popular discourses and seeking alternatives. Some of those alternative messages, such as "fuck cancer" have even gained a more mainstream position in the discourse.

Still, others don't receive them or opt out of such messages—or make their own. In some ways, our participants reify familiar illness narrative tropes that Arthur Frank (1995) identified; there are implied stories of restitution, chaos, and quest. But just as Frank makes it clear that illness stories are not merely stories, that their existence has larger and more profound social resonances, we found that the insights we could draw from talking with these women went further than unpacking how their breast cancer stories reveal depth. We could focus, instead, on how the health flashpoint itself gives way not to a narrative arc, but to a tornado of affect-laden rhetorical and meaning-making activity.

There are, of course, connections between a rhetorical community and a discourse community. Patients can transform from a member of a rhetorical community into a member of a discourse community when they accept their induction and immerse themselves in, for instance, the rhetoric of survivorship to find inspiration and meaning in their experience or else join a certain online support group that caters to their demographic or personal interests, such as a religion. When no discourse community exists, as many RHM studies have shown such as those in our previous work in *Women's Health Advocacy*, women are sometimes compelled to create one in order to share with other patients their own written materials, resources, and arguments where no rhetorical models existed—activities that we called "rhetorical ingenuity." Hence a rhetorical community is a complicated scene, and lest we step too close to describing its members in a passive role, the fluctuating connections between rhetorical encounters that are less than helpful and women's agitation that lead them to create their own messages and materials for a community together support our claim that epistemological consequences occur in rhetorical encounters and hence result in deliberative, internal and external processes that shape meaning, identity, and other important human facets.

Extending from our previous work in women's rhetorical ingenuity, the evidence in this study has helped us articulate these concepts and expand our thinking about patients in two ways: the first is our conception of patients as a greater, less defined/able rhetorical community. Considering patients this way allows for the summation of their experiences to be considered a nomos—*a set of agreed-upon terms of engagement* determined through experience in a community. Nomos is a sophistic-era approach to *coming to terms* (and not force) in order to make community decisions. Steven Pedersen (2017) has succinctly defined nomos as "socially-constructed beliefs and norms" (p. 6), and Susan Jarratt's (1991) resuscitation of the term for feminist rhetorical study affords credence to nomos as a way to consider language use as a middle-ground or feminist third space in service of creating deliberative communities and maintaining members' well-being (p. 48). In this study, nomos flows from patients' perspectives on the discourses surrounding and affecting them, a "middle ground" between patients' narratives (aligned with mythos) and patient education materials (aligned with logos).

To explore this middle ground, we have shifted our methodological attention away from patients' stories and experiences to their layered and deliberate engagements with the materials, resources, forms of support, and language use aimed at them. Many of the materials, resources, and supportive aspects of caretaking for cancer patients are rarely developed within a process of patient feedback or input (Melonçon, 2017). In fact, though many critiques of various medical and popular discourses around illnesses and especially breast cancer exist, fewer empirical studies exist around patients' reactions and experiences with PEM and other resources. One notable exception can be found in Kelly Pender's (2018) use of the voices of BRCA+ women she interviewed to develop a "rhetoric of care" that seeks to sidestep some of the constraints of exclusively biomedical accounts of what it means to be at genetic risk. Our work expands on Pender's by looking at the effects of the discourses surrounding breast cancer on patients and other health flashpoints in terms of their meaning-making.

From this project in epistemology, we have learned how women construe themselves as inductees into, particularly, breast cancer, menopause, and sobriety rhetorical communities. Patients take this invitation up variously, as our study and our own experiences show. This epistemology work is recognizable through patients' reactions, responses, rejections, alterations, and clap-backs to the messages and materials they encounter. Their telling of these reactions and responses—as well as our own observation and experience as women with health and medical experiences—inform a *nomos*, or community-derived terms of engagement wrought from experience that can and should influence each patient's local community, including doctors, friends, families, and caretakers which will hence expand existing supportive rhetorics. While, in this book, we focus on breast cancer, menopause, and sobriety as loci of rhetorical encounters, we believe the theory we present as a result of our findings can be usefully extended to most patient groups.

Joining the conversation: patient-centered research on patient support and materials

Medical scholarship has increasingly turned its eye to patient care and outcomes assessment stemming from patient-centered practices. This means that practitioners and researchers are producing studies that look at patient support as a means to patient empowerment with the goal of better clinical outcomes. However, numerous studies have found that most people do not take advantage of traditional face-to-face support groups: "Patients may not participate because of inconvenient meeting times, transportation and childcare issues, perception that their needs are not being specifically addressed, or reluctance to share their feelings or stories in public" (Attai et al., 2015, p. 2). So what kind of support, then, do patients want or need, and what kinds of support are most effective in helping patients make meaning from their illness?

We found that relatively few studies were looking at these questions, while some come near to the issue at hand. Scholarship focuses on the efficacy of PEM, systems of patient support provided in clinical settings, and in particular, the focus group as the main type of support, as well as the efficacy of support (again, typically support groups) on treatment efficacy. For instance, Chieh-Liang Wu et al. (2020) report on results of a three-year quality improvement study of patient support groups (PSGs) across a variety of illnesses (p. 5) in a hospital in Taiwan, noting that "engagement in PSGs is surprisingly low" (p. 2); they cite a study indicating that only 9.6% of patients participate in face-to-face support groups, while 4.4% participate in online support groups (p. 2).

Their focus, in both methods and discussion, is on developing a process that aims to improve PSGs. They indicate that "the values of PSGs include patient education, sharing experience, peer support, decreasing anxiety, improving quality of life, improvement of medication adherence, and building-up of the doctor–patient relationship" (p. 9). In the end, they found that their improvement process did work to improve the quality of PSGs (p. 11), but they do not consider patient desires in relation to PSGs or any support beyond PSGs.

Deanna Attai et al. (2015) studied a Twitter support group, surveying just over 200 women who used the hashtag #BCSM (breast cancer social media), which also has a blog, Facebook page, and weekly chat. They found that "breast cancer patients' perceived knowledge increases and their anxiety decreases by participation" (p. 1). They report that despite the low use of traditional peer-to-peer support groups (those that happen in person), "Social media is user-friendly and popular for health care consumers as evidenced by its rapid growth" (p. 3). Nevertheless, they find that social media support cannot replace face-to-face support:

> Twitter and other forms of social media cannot replace traditional office- and hospital-based resources for education and emotional support. In our survey, nearly 1 in 5 Twitter participants reported no improvement in education and 9% had persistent high anxiety despite #BCSM suggesting that Twitter participation was not sufficient to address education and anxiety needs in these patients. Therefore, the role of social media is to complement but not replace current practice.
>
> (p. 4)

Saira Hameed et al. (2018) also studied patient support groups; their participant pool included post-bariatric surgery patients. The study sought primarily to determine why people may have wanted support and what kind of support they needed. They hypothesized that patients with unfavorable outcomes (in this case, low weight loss or weight regain) would be most likely to want a peer support group (p. 2). This proved incorrect, and instead it was found that those who were struggling to keep weight off (but still managing to do so) were the ones who most wanted a support group (p. 5). They found that, "the most common request (from 65% respondents) was for educational sessions in the form of seminars and talks across a range of subject matters related to weight loss surgery" (p. 3). Importantly, they found that:

> Patients requested support in three areas: firstly, they wanted formal education delivered by experts about obesity, nutrition, exercise, and the weight loss surgery itself; secondly, they were looking for moral support from others who had experienced a similar journey; and thirdly, they expressed a desire to be able to keep in contact with professionals with a specialist interest in obesity should the need arise.
>
> (p. 5)

Outside of support group studies, Paul Bennett et al. (2018) report on a synthesis of studies relating to peer mentoring of patients with end stage kidney disease or those beginning dialysis. They assert that peer mentoring is more effective than "advice, education, and information from healthcare professionals who have not experienced kidney failure themselves, and thus, may not fully comprehend the challenges that each individual patient faces" (p. 455). Unlike clinicians, peer mentors "better relate and understand these challenges because they have lived through them and therefore are more 'expert' through their patient experience" (p. 455). Bennett et al. also found that:

> The more personal the education and information is, the more likely it is that people will make major changes in their lives and initiate (or improve) positive self-management in chronic disease. The notion of peers providing information and support to other peers may result in higher self-efficacy, given the source of the information: the peer "patient expert."
>
> (p. 455)

They conclude that "the benefits of peer mentor programs in dialysis include improved goal setting, improved decision-making, and self-management" at a stressful time (p. 460).

Judy King et al. (2019) also move beyond patient support groups; they examined how critical care patients' support needs changed as they transitioned from intensive care to home. They define "support needs" more broadly than a support group, as "additional help some adults need in order that they can live in the best way they can, despite any illness or disability they might have" (p. 2). They divided these needs into four categories: informational ("repeated transfer of clear, easily understandable information from healthcare staff to patients and families") (p. 4), emotional ("Needs expressed during the early initial stages included the need for comfort in words and touch and the support of family. The need for family support and attendance extended across time") (p. 7), instrumental needs ("personal care, hygiene and comfort, particularly relating to bathing, nutrition and pain relief") (p. 8), and appraisal ("Following ICU discharge, patients could appraise how far they had come") (p. 9). Of interest to our study:

> Patients stated they benefited from meeting others who had been through the ICU experience and understood the challenges they were addressing. They expressed an overwhelming desire to know that what they experienced was "normal," and that it took a long time and should not be concerned with slow progress. Patients gained comfort from identifying with others' experiences, and this helped normalise their own experiences.
>
> (p. 9)

Finally, studies of patient reported outcome measures (PROMs) seek to understand what type of support patients want, but researchers often pre-define the options, which is where qualitative study expands the field. Hameed et al. (2018) explain:

> PROMs are widely used to capture an individual patient's experience of their situation which might be different from that of their caregiver. PROM data allows for the patient's perspective to inform how healthcare is delivered and [...] what patients themselves want from a postoperative support group.
>
> (p. 2)

Joanne Greenhalgh et al. (2018) synthesized research aimed at showing how PROMs improve communication between patient and clinicians, showing that "the ways in which clinicians use PROMs is shaped by their relationships with patients and professional roles and boundaries" (p. 1).

Relevant to our project here, their research found that "PROMs completion prompts patients to reflect on their health and in doing so, patients develop a deeper understanding of how their condition affects them" (p. 22). Greenhalgh et al. (2018) continue, "the ways in which patients interpret questions and construct their answers is shaped by social and cultural factors and can affect the ways in which patients understand, frame or think about their condition" (p. 22). Further:

> PROMs ask "genuine questions," that is, questions which open up inquiry into the subject matter at hand but also the meaning of that subject matter. In order to answer a PROM item, respondents must infer both the subject matter of the question and the meaning of the subject matter implied by the question.
>
> (p. 22)

PROMs appear to have an interest in facilitating in patients an epistemological process in which they create meaning from/about their illness.

Our research picks up the mantle to understand that process itself, although our participants and selves were not participants in a PROM study. Our definition for patient support is much broader than clinical studies and ask of our participants: who and what within your support network of people helped you navigate information, rhetorical work, experience emotions, make decisions, and ultimately make meaning of your illness or health flashpoint, with the assumption that the process demands different needs and inputs during its various phases and especially outside of the clinic?

Methodology

As is clear, at the outset of this project, we were, at base, interested in how patients use rhetoric (conceived broadly) to navigate the various options available to them when they are faced with a new health flashpoint—including having a strong desire to learn more about the roles affect, support, and helpful or harmful information play in such processes. Methodologically, then, we rely on an adaptation of multiple ontologies as a way to examine and highlight the sources of information and forms of support that might be beneficial. That is, we think about the many overlapping, everyday forms of being that can become integral, everyday rhetorical elements of a person's attempts to patch together a livable life as they are contending with alarming diagnoses, punishing courses of treatment, and opacous next chapters. We argue that these often affect-laden and blurry rhetorical practices constitute an episteme. In this way, we rely on Mol's (2002) work as it is adapted by Pender (2018) in which Pender asks readers to think about "what it is that patients do in order to live a good life when what they really want—perfect health—is not possible" (p. 21). Each chapter engages in an investigation that is more diffuse than typical studies of patient education materials that examine things like readability, yet we do retain a clear focus on how everyday patients navigate information and support.

With this orientation in mind, the methods are four-fold and include survey data, focus group data, textual analysis, and rhetorical autoethnography, each of which will be further explicated and grounded in the context of the participants' experiences, our experiences, and in each discourse arena of women's health flashpoints including breast cancer, menopause, and sobriety in the following chapters.

Chapter summaries

Following this introductory chapter, Chapter 2 offers a more detailed explanation of our theory of the process of patient epistemology in which we unpack our terms, share our graphic model of the process itself, and explicate the reasons why such a process should be articulated.

Chapter 3 then takes up how women who have experienced the health flashpoints of breast cancer diagnosis, treatment, and aftercare have found meaning and support through the constitutive rhetorical work embedded throughout. Such that we could learn more about this topic, we conducted initial survey research to examine the sources of information and forms of support that breast cancer patients and survivors find generative and helpful versus stagnating and hurtful. We, then, arranged focus groups as a way to gather more granular information on specific experiences women have had with both sources of information and forms of support. Relying primarily on an analysis of that focus group data, the chapter ultimately shares how our theory of patient epistemologies was developed.

Chapter 4 turns to the health flashpoint of menopause or, more precisely, perimenopausal symptoms that eventually lead to the full cessation of menses, or menopause. Methodologically, we perform critical discourse analysis on a corpus of public-facing texts about this topic, grounded in *doxa*, to argue that women experiencing the health flashpoints of perimenopause and menopause will find decades-worth of a consistent, cyclical claim: that women do not have adequate information about menopause, its symptoms, or potential treatment, nor do they have any real support to manage this daunting transitional space. This reiteration, we argue, leads to inertia under the guise of newness. Subsequently, fewer attempts at unpacking why perimenopause and menopause are so difficult are offered. All of the discursive space is taken up already by the popular opinion that there is simply insufficient information. For us, though, too many arguments that claim that lack of information is to blame for menopause being an unpleasant and unsupported phase of life take attention away from the real culprit—misogyny, and especially abject hatred of older and aging women—a well-documented cultural phenomenon that is nonetheless too rarely equated with this health flashpoint (Åberg et al., 2020; Chrisler, 2011; Nosek et al., 2010; Syme & Cohn, 2016).

In Chapter 5, we continue to show how the processes of patient epistemologies are either helped along or hindered within a rhetorical community through the case of the health flashpoint of seeking sobriety or coming to terms with disordered substance use. Alcoholism and its discourses have long been dominated, as many readers know, by the traditions and habits of Alcoholics Anonymous (AA) and the attendant widely used Twelve Steps, which are present not only in the non-expert terrain of sobriety treatment but also in various popular and professional settings. Likewise, the discourse of AA has already been thoroughly taken to task for being exclusionary and myopic in its male-centric and overtly Christian ethos. The chapter is not, then, another attempt to revamp and assuage these elements of AA discourse for a female audience. Since such female-centric versions of AA and the Twelve Steps already exist, we, instead, show how they do not always deliver on the promise of displacing the problematic elements therein, and we show the kinds of paradigm shifts that can impact addiction treatment and alter the cycle of patient epistemologies in a helpful way.

Chapter 6 presents a more fully articulated version of the cycle of patient epistemologies by zooming in on a specific set of health flashpoints in one person's life. In Chapter 6, then, Bryna presents an autoethnographic account of the various health flashpoints that have constituted her own experiences with breast cancer diagnoses, treatment, aftercare, and beyond.

Finally, in Chapter 7, we summarize the contributions of this book; namely, tracked through a variety of health conditions and realities, this book has helped to better articulate the sources of information and forms of support that help women through the often-daunting rhetorical work that goes along with life-changing health flashpoints. While some may experience long stretches of wellness, most of us will, instead, experience some periods of wellness that are interspersed with illness, injuries, or other medical or health-related crises that alter our affective, cognitive, and material landscapes forever.

Our audience

We see two main audiences for this book and theory. The first is constituted by the academic communities to which we belong and wish to contribute in service of ever-expanding and useful Rhetorics of Health and Medicine. Additionally, we also see practical advice in this book for a certain set of people. To be clear: It is not our purpose to offer advice about the *what* of coping with illness—it is not about how or whether to choose a flat closure after a mastectomy or about the benefits or dangers of hormone replacement therapy, although our study supports that an important part of making those kinds of decisions are other women's stories and experiences. The book does feature examples of women making these types of decisions and narrating the difficulties of doing so. But it is pointedly not a book for only patients; it is instead a book for friends, for family members, for spouses, for care providers, caretakers, and others in supportive roles in order for them to become (more) aware of the crowded rhetorical field a patient enters into when they receive a diagnosis and the many complicated and usually overwhelming and sometimes infuriating discursive acts and epistemological processes they will undergo alongside the physical challenge of illness and treatment. This is what Fassin (2018), about whose work we will presently share more, calls a clash of their biography and biology. We asked women to tell us (and thought about ourselves) what kinds of things—messages, information, suggestions, and offers—were most helpful and supportive to them during diagnosis, treatment, and aftercare because we think the importance and effects of these on the illness experience are under-studied or under-appreciated.

Therefore, given our new understanding of the process at work, we hope that caretakers and support people will be better able to offer appropriate support that will afford patients a measure of agency and clear the way for the important and usually difficult, rhetorical work that, in the 21st century medical-industrial complex, must accompany the physical, emotional, and practical difficulties of illness. Among and between these rhetorical acts swirl emotion and identity-formation, which together constitute and contribute to the many ways patients make meaning.

References

Åberg, E., Kukkonen, I., & Sarpila, O. (2020). From double to triple standards of aging: Perceptions of physical appearance at the intersections of age, gender and class. *Journal of Aging Studies, 55.* https://doi.org/10.1016/j.jaging.2020.100876

Attai, D. J., Cowher, M. S., Al-Hamadani, M., Schoger, J. M., Staley, A. C., & Landercasper, J. (2015). Twitter social media is an effective tool for breast cancer patient education and support: Patient-reported outcomes by survey. *Journal of Medical Internet Research, 17*(7). https://doi.org/10.2196/jmir.4721

Bennett, P. N., St. Clair Russell, J., Atwal, J., Brown, L., & Schiller, B. (2018). Patient-to-patient peer mentor support in dialysis: Improving the patient experience. *Seminars in Dialysis, 31*(5), 455–461. https://doi.org/10.1111/sdi.12703

Chrisler, J. C. (2011). Leaks, lumps, and lines: Stigma and women's bodies. *Psychology of Women Quarterly, 35*(2), 202–214. https://doi.org/10.1177/0361684310397698

Fassin, D. (2018). *Life: A critical user's manual.* Polity Press.

Frank, A. (1995). *The wounded storyteller: Body, illness, and ethics.* University of Chicago Press.

Greenhalgh, J., Gooding, K., Gibbons, E., Dalkin, S., Wright, J., Valderas, J., & Black, N. (2018). How do patient reported outcome measures (PROMs) support clinician-patient communication and patient care? A realist synthesis. *Journal of Patient-Reported Outcomes, 2*(42), 1–28. https://doi.org/10.1186/s41687-018-0061-6

Hameed, S., Salem, V., Tan, T. M., Collins, A., Shah, K., Scholz, S., Ahmed, A. R., & Chahal, H. (2018). Beyond weight loss: Establishing a postbariatric surgery patient support group—What do patients want? *Journal of Obesity,* 1–7. https://doi.org/10.1155/2018/8419120

Jarratt, S. (1991). *Rereading the sophists: Classical rhetoric refigured.* Southern Illinois University Press.

Kessler, M. M. (2022). *Stigma stories: Rhetoric, lived experience, and chronic illness.* The Ohio State University Press.

King, J., O'Neill, B., Ramsay, P., Linden, M. A., Darweish Medniuk, A., Outtrim, J., & Blackwood, B. (2019). Identifying patients' support needs following critical illness: A scoping review of the qualitative literature. *Critical Care, 23*(1), 1–12. https://doi.org/10.1186/s13054-019-2441-6

Lipari, M., Berlie, H., Saleh, Y., Hang, P., & Moser, L. (2019). Understandability, actionability, and readability of online patient education materials about diabetes mellitus. *American Journal of Health-System Pharmacy, 76*(3), 182–186. https://doi.org/10.1093/ajhp/zxy021

Melonçon, L. K. (2017). Patient experience design: Expanding usability methodologies for healthcare. *Communication Design Quarterly, 5*(2), 19–28. https://doi.org/10.1145/3131201.3131203

Melonçon, L., & Scott, J. B. (2018). Manifesting a scholarly dwelling place in RHM. *Rhetoric of Health & Medicine, 1*(1–2), i–x. https://doi.org/10.5744/rhm.2018.1001

Mol, A. (2002). Cutting surgeons, walking patients: Some complexities involved in comparing. In J. Law & A. Mol (Eds.), *Complexities: Social studies of knowledge practices* (pp. 218–257). Duke University Press.

Nosek, M., Kennedy, H. P., Beyene, Y., Taylor, D., Gilliss, C., & Lee, K. (2010). The effects of perceived stress and attitudes toward menopause and aging on symptoms of menopause. *Journal of Midwifery and Women's Health, 55*(4), 328–334. https://doi.org/10.1016/j.jmwh.2009.09.005

Öresland, S., Friberg, F., Määttä, S., & Öhlen, J. (2015). Disclosing discourses: Biomedical and hospitality discourses in patient education materials. *Nursing Inquiry, 22*(3), 240–248. https://doi.org/10.1111/nin.12097

Pedersen, S. M. (2017). A composed "rhetoric" in place: A material-epistemic reading of Plato's Phaedrus. *Rhetoric Review, 36*(1), 1–14. https://doi.org/10.1080/07350198.2017.1245999

Pender, K. (2018). *Being at genetic risk: Toward a rhetoric of care.* University of Pennsylvania Press.

Reed, A. (2018). Building on bibliography: Toward useful categorization of research in rhetorics of health and medicine. *Journal of Technical Writing and Communication, 48*(2), 175–198. https://doi.org/10.1177/0047281616667904

16   *Starting from friendship and rhetoric*

Restaino, J. (2019). *Surrender: Feminist rhetoric and ethics in love and illness.* Southern Illinois University Press.

Reynolds, J. F. (2018). A short history of mental health rhetoric research (MHRR). *Rhetoric of Health & Medicine, 1*(1–2), 1–18. https://doi.org/10.5744/rhm.2018.1003

Segal, J. Z. (2008). Breast cancer narratives as public rhetoric: Genre itself and the maintenance of ignorance. *Linguistics and the Human Sciences, 3*(1), 3–23.

Syme, M. L., & Cohn, T. J. (2016). Examining aging sexual stigma attitudes among adults by gender, age, and generational status. *Aging and Mental Health, 20*(1), 36–45. https://doi.org/10.1080/13607863.2015.1012044

Whitaker, H. (2021). *Quit like a woman: The radical choice to not drink in a culture obsessed with alcohol.* Random House Publishing Group.

Wu, C. L., Liou, C. H., Chen, C. H., Sheu, W. H., Chou, I. J., & Tsai, S. F. (2020). Quality improvement initiatives in reforming patient support groups—Three-year outcomes. *International Journal of Environmental Research and Public Health, 17*(19). https://doi.org/10.3390/ijerph17197155

2 Toward a theory of patient epistemologies

How health flashpoints engender cyclical rhetorical and identity work

In 2018's *Life: A Critical User's Manual*, Didier Fassin drew on a number of philosophic and social scientific texts to account for the problematic disentanglement of biographical life from biological life (or of experience from matter) as it plays out across disciplinary boundaries. Theorizing a blending of the two via his own empirical studies alongside a meditation on a number of philosophic texts, he presented a reflection on the enmeshing and overlaps that better account for how human life unfolds. Fassin concluded that when naturalist and humanist approaches are examined as co-mingled entities, the ethical landscape of human life reveals troubling inequities. As we attempt to describe the rhetorical and identity-shaping work that patients undertake at the onset, during, and after a health crisis or flashpoint such that they might make meaning of their experience, we see resonances with Fassin's work. Part of what happens when a person encounters such a flashpoint is that they are jolted by the incommensurability of their immediate biological life and their biographical life as they've always known, or at least imagined it. The health flashpoint creates a disruption, that is, in the person's very real physical body, and that interruption does more than change the physicality of the person. It also very much changes the subjective experience of being a specific person with a history and an envisioned future living at a specific point in space and time. Similarly, Michael Bury's (1982) frequently cited work on chronic illness as biographical disruption used interviews with rheumatoid arthritis patients to show how disruptions in biography are "at one and the same time, disruptions of social relationships and the ability to mobilize material resources" (p. 180).

Just as Fassin compellingly showed how biological life and biographical life are often conceived of separately, we theorize that health flashpoints are essentially a person's physical body colliding with their sense of self. Fassin's text allows us to meditate on an interruption that erupts at the level of biological and biographical life. That is, while biological life is always there, of course, it is also sometimes too easy to ignore it, particularly in the day-to-day, neoliberally mandated hyper-productive schedules that most of us operate under. In health crises, the biological asserts itself and comes roaring back into focus, throwing the biographical features of life into disarray. Health

DOI: 10.4324/9781003398318-2

flashpoints, in this way, present moments when a person's biological life and biographical life collide. In many ways, life, as the person had been living it in the day-to-day, ceases to exist, and simultaneously, the story a person knows and tells about their life takes on new meanings and directions. The process is painful since a person has a sense of their history, a story, and ideas about a future that is shifting beneath their feet. We contend that it requires extraordinary rhetorical work to begin to reconcile the new meanings and directions— even as we also acknowledge that, depending on the severity of the health flashpoint, the biological body may not really be ignorable in the same ways that it might've been before. Thus, part of what we mean by "patients making meaning" and "patient epistemologies" is the stitching together of the biological and the biographical, and in the best cases, emerging a bit more mindful in terms of what it means to live in a body that is constantly in a state of deterioration in one way or another. Additionally, the body is part of a larger *body politic* that must contend with various socioeconomic and material forces and limitations. The rhetorical work enmeshed in health flashpoints often requires sitting with and being with this feeling that the body is constantly declining, which is incommensurate with how most of us live, even as disability study scholars have for time immemorial been urging us all to consider ourselves as temporarily able-bodied or able-minded, if we were ever fully able-bodied or able-minded to begin with.[1]

Reconciling new biological realities with a biographical life as it has been known is excessively difficult and complex work, and our theoretical attempts to unpack some of that complexity begins by asking: how is that reconciling done? We posit that the cycle of patient epistemologies is one articulation of what happens as a person undergoes this difficult work. In the midst of this disjunction that occurs between biological life and biographical life that a health flashpoint presents, a theory of patient epistemologies is necessary to reflect and articulate the many complex factors that drive the rhetorical/ epistemological work that goes into not only facing but even shaping a new reality, as well as the many steps or forms of cognitive effort that work takes.

By complex factors, we mean a person's subjectivities, histories, emotions, material conditions, support networks, and educational level—all of the pieces and parts of their biographical life as they come into contact with biological life. And by rhetorical and identity work, we are emphasizing the often hidden or taken-for-granted level of meaning-making that patients undertake during health crises that derives from reading, writing, discussing, deliberating, risk-weighing, and decision-making—all implicitly rhetorical activities. As such, our participants' and our own health experiences as inductees into often unwanted rhetorical communities have taught us that the health realities and problems or diseases we suffer from and the treatments that may be assumed to be a person's central focus during a health crisis very often compete for attention and co-mingle with this rhetorical and identity work. There are many examples of the effects of this competition and co-mingling, including affective factors such as increased stress, anger, and other emotions, as well as gaps in care and support that have been of interest to those who study the rhetoric of health and medicine (RHM) and which our study has sought to also illuminate and describe.

In fact, our theory of patient epistemologies seeks to add to the expanding field of RHM. While inquiries into health and medical topics using rhetorical theories predate the use of the term RHM, the field represents the relatively recent, conscious efforts of scholars to bring together threads of research that use rhetorical theories with a wide variety of social scientific and humanistic methodological approaches to aid in researchers finding existing work (Eberhard, 2012; Lynch & Zoller, 2015; Melonçon & Frost, 2015; Reed, 2018; Scott et al., 2013). Scholarship in RHM is extremely heterogeneous and ranges from conceptual and theoretical (Campbell & Angeli, 2019; Derkatch, 2016; Edwell, 2017; Graham et al., 2018; Hite & Carter, 2019; Kessler, 2020; Larson, 2021; Pender, 2018; Presley, 2021; Sánchez, 2020) to pragmatic and applied (Barton, 2004, 2007; Campbell, 2018; Davis & Dubisar, 2019; Kuehl et al., 2020; Longtin & Binion, 2021; Ryan, 2021; Swacha & St.Amant, 2021; Welhausen, 2015; Welhausen & Bivens, 2022; Burnett et al., 2013) with various permutations in between.

While early texts spent a good deal of time delineating permeable boundaries for the field and describing various possibilities for methodological approaches (Angeli & Johnson-Sheehan, 2018; Gouge, 2018; Hannah & Arduser, 2018; Melonçon & Scott, 2017, 2018; Molloy et al., 2018; Scott et al., 2013), and work in the intervening years used those foundational/definitional texts to add to a growing corpus of work in a number of topics, newer work has moved into more explicitly activist territory via, and, among other things, engagement with antiracist movements such as, for example, reproductive justice (Harper, 2020; Novotny et al., 2020; Novotny & Hertogh, 2022), collaborations with disability studies (Holladay, 2017), and crossovers with scientific and technical communication discourses (Angeli, 2015; Angeli, 2019; Welhausen & Bivens, 2022). Like other fields of academic study, RHM has been, in recent years, reevaluated in terms of tendencies toward myopia, ingroup thinking, and white supremacy (Dutta, 2022; Sastry et al., 2021). These critiques arrived in the midst of and energized efforts at increasing inclusivity, such as amplifying the work in related areas such as reproductive justice cited above, and those efforts have intensified (Joyner et al., 2023; Molloy & Hensley Owens, 2022; Scott et al., 2021).

This book contributes to such efforts in RHM by explicitly addressing marginalized positionalities across conditions in each of the data chapters, by putting forward a versatile theoretical approach that will aid in future patient-centered work, and by focusing on the information and support that help or hinder cycles of patient epistemologies—crucial processes to unpack in the work of creating more equitable health futures.

Blending humanistic and social scientific modes of inquiry that converge in rhetorical theories, we add to the field's interest in theory-building

(Melonçon & Scott, 2017). While many excellent RHM projects focus on a single health or medical phenomenon or ailment (Arduser, 2017; Bennett, 2019; Pender, 2018), this book uses several health and medical examples to build out a theory that could be useful across even more issues and topics. While each chapter is an attempt to offer a practical takeaway for a range of stakeholders, the project, as a whole, makes an important methodological and theoretical intervention into the field by offering a way to describe patients' engagements with sources of information and forms of support beyond readability and finding community.

In describing the process of epistemology, or meaning-making derived from rhetorical and identity work, we hold space for the many elements at play, including:

- the patient, with all their various and unique social, material, bodily, emotional, mental, family circumstances, backgrounds, and truths
- the social contexts in which persons experience their health flashpoints, as well as their gender, sexuality, race, ethnicity, religion, education, socioeconomic status, and family background
- emotions and affective responses that may or may not conform to the dominant modes of emotions that are often held up as values during illness, such as positivity and resolve
- care conditions within a huge range from ideal to injurious, including emotional support from others; physical help with tasks, driving, and other duties; comfortable space; and competing interests (e.g., household needs)
- Iterations of health flashpoints over the course of the lifespan, or how health experiences overlap, compound, and interact with each other

We see these elements as constitutive of an epistemological process that includes "steps" or sets of experiences that occur in an iterative pattern that we have observed based on our participants' and our own experiences. These include

- the health flashpoint itself, which can bring in fear, shock, confusion, and physical and emotional pain, and is often unable to be extracted as a standalone experience. It is bound up, as "health news" always is, in medical and other discourses that shape understandings upon delivery
- the rhetorical encounter, or sometimes head-long collision with collections of discourses associated with and creating the reality of a particular realm of disease, condition, or treatment. For an example drawn from our study, entering at least partially indeterminate states of being such as perimenopause also means entering a decades-long discursively shaped reality which paints the experience of menopause as no different for women in 2022 than it was in 1990

- rhetorical work, including looking for and reading information (or sometimes actively ignoring information on purpose out of fear or denial), thinking, weighing options, recapitulating and synthesizing information that has been gathered from various sources, passive and agentive decision-making, and devising systems to share information with others
- reflection, which includes time, purposeful attempts to ponder, accidental realizations and learning, talking with others (whether professionals, other patients, or loved ones), as well as writing, which Bryna's autoethnography in Chapter 6 exhibits well as a unique contribution to the literature on patient experience

While these have, in our experiences and in the lives of our participants, loosely unfolded in order, they also often overlap and collapse in on one another more than they have neat starts and stops of their own.

How persons make meaning because of and during a health flashpoint has loomed large in our and our participants' lives when contending with health problems, and our analyses of health discourses have helped us describe what has happened to us and other women, rhetorically, affectively, in terms of identity, and materially-speaking during these events. However, meaning-making is forged by an ever-unique interplay between the above-noted elements. There is not only one way to observe, understand, or characterize how it occurs, but it does occur, and its results offer the best sense of "proof" of the importance of this process. This process is undoubtedly worth further consideration and development on a granular level as the new theory we are proposing here has broad applicability across contexts and around the globe.

For example, in sub-Saharan Africa, HIV testing is not always performed in a timely manner (Tetteh et al., 2022), yet a theory of patient epistemologies that took seriously the disruption in biographical and biological life and how that relates to affect, overwhelm and a person's willingness to test could lead to stronger theories and interventions that could increase testing and, thus, appropriate care. In China, where instances of lung cancer are slated to continue to rise (Fang et al., 2022), a theory of patient epistemologies could prove useful when determining the most appropriate variety of patient education materials and social supports for the newly diagnosed. Even considering large-scale conflict and natural disasters as constituting communal health flashpoints could help to illuminate how communities work through attendant life-altering public health emergencies on the whole and how individuals contend with such catastrophes in their own lives. Likewise, pandemics and epidemics could be usefully theorized as health flashpoints with global ramifications wherein cycles of patient epistemologies could be a useful theoretical frame to unpack how specific populations make sense of what is going on, receive and understand information, and recuperate their lives and senses of self.

Indeed, living in bodies in constant states of deterioration and aging is an irrefutable part of every human being's life. The interplay of elements in the iterative and often recursive cycle of patient epistemologies results in major life decisions, in body changes, and in changes in mental health status. Such results have impermeably changed our and our participants' lives and senses of self, which in turn continue to contribute to identity-formation, physical and mental health, life decisions, relationships, everyday habits, and material circumstances, etc. even long after the immediate flashpoint subsides. While this book provides cases of the cycle of patient epistemologies and other meditations on how this theory works conceptually, we also seek to contribute a highly adaptable theoretical approach to looking at what happens to an individual person or communities when they face a new health flashpoint such that other scholars across disciplines interested in how human beings create new meaning from health experiences might use our framework in their own analyses.

Therefore, the chief result and claim of our study is a process theory of patient epistemology, which is presented graphically in Figure 2.1. The following is a narrative explanation that takes up each element in turn and situates it within and among its constituent counterparts to represent our ideation of this process. Each patient and person will be able to identify and tailor "how" this meaning-making experience stemming from a health flashpoint occurs or occurred for them.

We also contend that a support or care person for a patient can look to this process and think about "where" they fit into it by considering, perhaps for the first time, how meaningful both intended and unintended said and unsaid discourse, messages, and forms of support are within such a complicated and high-stakes process. That is, a process theory of patient epistemologies has pragmatic value for those whose loved ones, friends, or neighbors are facing new health circumstances as it can help to illuminate the forms of support

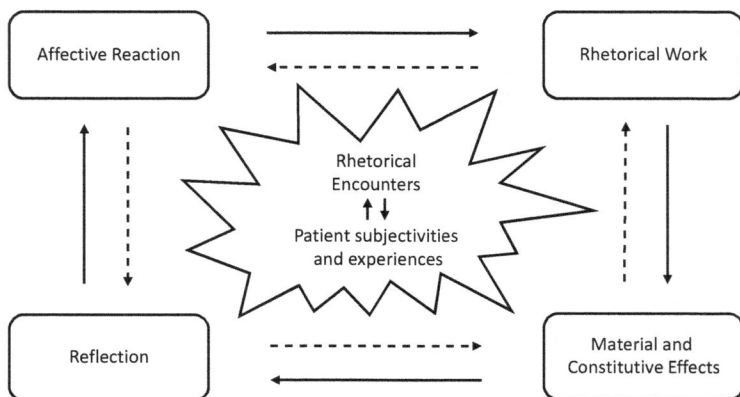

Figure 2.1 A process theory of patient epistemology

that would be helpful and welcome versus the attempts at support that might, instead, be detrimental and unwelcome.

Health flashpoints begin our conception of patient epistemology, especially when a diagnosis or health problem or change disrupts a person's life, scares them, and/or causes them pain. The health flashpoint usually co-mingles with an onslaught of discourses that a person is likely to encounter upon delivery of health news. Often chiefly medical, discourses will inevitably be interpretable and make effects through the terministic screens of the unique person's subjectivities, experiences, and specific social and material contexts. In addition, the patient reacts, responds, uptakes, or perhaps ignores these discourses, but these discourses are bound to shape the reality of the health concern and sense of self along with an affective response.

We term exposure to discourses within a health flashpoint as "rhetorical encounters." The word "encounter" is chosen to highlight the uninvited, unplanned, and even sometimes accidental nature of learning one's diagnosis, or being made aware of a health problem or change. Encounters are often immediate and overwhelming, sometimes agnotological or antiquated and therefore actually unhelpful. Discourses are mostly often medical, but by way of discussing one's health flashpoint with nearly anyone in one's life, a patient can encounter discourses that are cultural, professional, and sometimes amateur. An important point is that health flashpoints are never not embroiled in language and discourse that shapes a person's understanding and experience simultaneously, and they offer available epistemological frameworks, often culturally approved stock narratives, which, when critiqued through feminist lenses, reveal rootedness in patriarchy and misogyny. Health flashpoints often have epistemological frameworks built right in, as our chapters on menopause and sobriety will evidence.

Experiencing a health flashpoint and its inevitable rhetorical encounters results in many emotions, fears, and causes for alarm. In our configuration of the cycle of patient epistemologies, we hold space for the affective in the rhetoric of health and medicine since, often, emotions are not acknowledged as part of the patient experience beyond perhaps information on how care providers should allow space for and "handle" patient affect when, in contrast, affective responses are probably the chief concern second only to physical discomfort or pain when people are experiencing a health flashpoint. Specifically, patients who must undertake rhetorical work, such as deliberating possibilities and making decisions, often allow and indeed prioritize emotions when making decisions, something our participants and personal experiences have brought to the fore in this epistemological process.

As we also found, emotions very much influence the way patients seek out, avoid, sort, and understand forms of information related to their new health realities. For instance, a person with a new cancer diagnosis may find themselves so overwhelmed and fearful of their chances of dying that they would restrict the information and websites they allowed themselves to visit since some sites, they reason, may exacerbate that fear—a behavior we heard described in our breast cancer focus groups. On the other hand, other women casted around quite a bit to find useful information from real people, not just the well-known, antiseptic websites such as WebMD. As another example of the layers of rhetorical work occurring and how emotions play a role, Bryna recognized that repeating and telling sad news or complicated medical information was going to wear her down over time; she set up a private Facebook group to make her reports, avoiding repeated phone calls or singular texts to many people.

Emotions and affective responses, the cycle of patient epistemologies as we conceive it, need more room in studies of health and rhetoric—not only do our participants (and we) have important stories to tell, but they register/ed emotions that are often overshadowed by a powerful public imperative that patients, for their own good, must demonstrate determination, bravery, and other watchwords of stock health narratives in which a neat narrative arc unfolds from diagnosis to treatment to wellness—all marked by extreme bravery and grit. We believe it should go without saying that such arcs leave out the vast majority of people facing health crises. Instead, our model centers the fact that patients are shocked, sad, scared, overwhelmed, frustrated, misunderstood, and angry. It is important to account for these emotions in studies of rhetorical circumstances such as health flashpoints, lest we assume that the range of rhetorical work involved in patient epistemology is done in less complicated contexts.

Next, alongside and within this process is ongoing rhetorical activity that includes reading, listening, sorting, reasoning, discussing, questioning, making decisions, etc. that yield both material and constitutive, identity-forming effects. The rhetorical activity, we have explained, is influenced by the affective, unpleasant, and emotional difficulty of these life choices, including anger, fear, and regret. Although rhetorical work is depicted in a box, a great deal of activity and tension must be imagined during this portion of the experience/process. As we allude to above, women in our study reported rhetorical work such as finding information, choosing how it is consumed, reading and researching, decision-making, communicating with family and support people, trying to explain things to children without too much alarm, having to file and organize information, joining communities online, avoiding certain topics or rabbit holes, "telling their story" (usually argued as empowering), or making decisions about accepting or rejecting mainstream narratives and metaphors.

This part of the cycle co-mingles with material and constitutive effects, meaning that emotions' bearing on rhetorical work can result in a prioritization of the biographical part of life during a health crisis. For instance, our participant Leslie, about whom the reader will learn more in the next chapter, chose to delay her first round of breast cancer treatments until after her six-year-old daughter's birthday, a decision that on its face may seem irrational and unsafe, but which illustrates how emotions and identities loom large in the process. Leslie's identity as a mother and provider of stability for her daughter played perhaps an outsized role in her decision-making, depending on how you look at it. We cannot calculate the material effects of Leslie's decision, but we can see that Leslie was determined to maintain her biographical sense of herself if just for a month before she further grappled with her biological needs.

This step in the process is an apt instance in which to explain the arrows in our cycle; note that the bold arrows go clockwise from step to step in order to illustrate the general nature of the cycle as we are able to describe it based on our observations of our participants, our own experiences, and the discourses we have analyzed. However, note that the dotted arrows go counter-clockwise alongside the others. This graphic representation is meant to highlight the ways that these steps can back-track or occur out of order, or capitulate between two before moving on (or back) to another step. Between the affective, rhetorical, and material and constitutive effects, another example provides more understanding of the nature of these elements. Bryna, during her health flashpoint of her second instance of breast cancer in 2020, was faced with and forced to worry about a tree on her property becoming unsafe. In the midst of handling an annoying but not otherwise impossible household responsibility, her anger, confusion, and sense of absurdity about her own life—examples of the affective and the constitutive—spiked and preoccupied her, making her material life even harder to deal with than it would otherwise have been. Given that she was mid-health scare and spending her time tracking down property maps, calling the city, and booking a tree service, she was thrust into an epistemological cycle. These instances of hard-to-trace but real demands of human meaning-making within a health crisis evidence the need and potential power of a theory to understand them better.

Reflection is depicted at the end of this process, and we have observed that this step happens largely after the acute phase of an illness, rather than during it. That said, we want to emphasize that this step does not occur immediately or on a schedule, and it, perhaps unsurprisingly, recapitulates in a person's life to shape and reshape their understandings as well as continued, revised, or new material and rhetorical action over time and perhaps for the rest of one's life.

It is in the reflection where the person attempts to reconcile their new biological realities with their biographical understandings of their own life spans. This point acknowledges the lived reality of all three of the health arenas in this book, with cancer affecting our participants' health generally and negatively even far after their completed treatments; the fact that perimenopause creates effects for the remainder of one's life after onset; and the fact that sobriety is an everyday choice and practice for the rest of one's life, should a person succeed in their sobriety. The reflection can look like many things and sometimes repeats to the rhetorical work stage—often, with some distance and time to encapsulate or come to new understandings of one's experience, women share their stories, their advice, become activists, or lead support groups for others. In a small way, our chapter on menopause offers this type of reflection and rhetorical action, as we critique and offer a new perspective on how women (like us) can and should add more dimensions to menopause discourses and expand the epistemological capacity of the support available to women who will enter menopause.

Even as we describe these stages and steps, we want to emphasize that, while it does often offer space for critique, theorizing patient epistemologies is not meant to be polemical or strictly critical of the sources of information and forms of support that exist across the health flashpoints we examine. Indeed, it is meant to offer space to think through how precisely a person comes to know themselves in the midst of their health experiences and how, therefore, they contend with the cyclical meaning-making that will ultimately drive crucial decision-making—decision-making that will impact not only their own bodies and persons but the people and communities around them.

In its attention to what a person brings to a health flashpoint (and vice-versa), inherent in a theory of patient epistemologies is an acknowledgment of the role that allostatic load (or the accumulation of maladies on the body that are the result of chronic stress) and social determinants of health (SDOH)— "the conditions in the environments where people are born, live, learn, work, play, worship, and age that affect a wide range of health, functioning, and quality-of-life outcomes and risks" (U.S. Department of Health and Human Services)—play in health and medical experiences and encounters. We believe our theory can function adjacent to, and in a way that very much complements these two powerful concepts in health as our theory offers more empirical information on how patients experience health and illness in their everyday lives. In the chapters that follow, we attempt to demonstrate the usefulness of this theory through an examination of specific conditions and then conclude with a longer meditation on our methodological approaches and how our theory can be adapted to other studies and circumstances around the globe.

Note

1   While "temporarily able-bodied" or "TAB" has been in use since at least the 1970s, recent disability scholars and activists have pointed out its limitations as it creates community while reinforcing disability stigmas.

References

Angeli, E. L. (2015). Three types of memory in emergency medical services communication. *Written Communication, 32*(1), 3–38.

Angeli, E. L. (2019). *Rhetorical work in emergency medical services: Communicating in the unpredictable workplace.* Routledge.

Angeli, E. L., & Johnson-Sheehan, R. (2018). Introduction to the special issue: Medical humanities and/or the rhetoric of health and medicine. *Technical Communication Quarterly*, 27(1), 1–6. https://doi.org/10.1080/10572252.2018.1399746

Arduser, L. (2017). *Living chronic: Agency and expertise in the rhetoric of diabetes*. The Ohio State University Press.

Barton, E. (2004). Discourse methods and critical practice in professional communication the front-stage and back-stage discourse of prognosis in medicine. *Journal of Business and Technical Communication*, 18(1), 67–111. https://doi.org/10.1177/1050651903258127

Barton, E. (2007). Commentary 3. Quality of life to the end. *Communication and Medicine*, 4(1), 121–123. https://doi.org/10.1515/CAM.2007.014

Bennett, J. (2019). *Managing diabetes: The cultural politics of disease*. NYU Press.

Burnett, R. E., Cooper, L. A., & Welhausen, C. A. (2013). What do technical communicators need to know about collaboration? In J. Johnson-Eilola & S. Selber (Eds.), *Solving problems in technical communication* (pp. 454–478). University of Chicago Press.

Bury, M. (1982). Chronic illness as biographical disruption. *Sociology of Health and Illness*, 4(2), 167–182. https://doi.org/10.1111/1467-9566.ep11339939

Campbell, L. (2018). The rhetoric of health and medicine as a "teaching subject": Lessons from the medical humanities and simulation pedagogy. *Technical Communication Quarterly*, 27(1), 7–20. https://doi.org/10.1080/10572252.2018.1401348

Campbell, L., & Angeli, E. L. (2019). Embodied healthcare intuition: A taxonomy of sensory cues used by healthcare providers. *Rhetoric of Health & Medicine*, 2(4), 353–383. https://muse.jhu.edu/pub/227/article/744859

Davis, S., & Dubisar, A. M. (2019). Communicating elective sterilization: A feminist perspective. *Rhetoric of Health & Medicine*, 2(1), 88–113. https://doi.org/10.5744/rhm.2019.1004

Derkatch, C. (2016). *Bounding biomedicine: Evidence and rhetoric in the new science of alternative medicine*. University of Chicago Press.

Dutta, M. J. (2022). The whiteness of the rhetoric of health and medicine (RHM): A culture-centered framework for dismantling. *Departures in Critical Qualitative Research*, 11(1–2), 54–79. https://doi.org/10.1525/dcqr.2022.11.1-2.54

Eberhard, J. (2012). An annotated bibliography of literature on the rhetoric of health and medicine. *Present Tense*, 2(2). https://www.presenttensejournal.org/volume-2/an-annotated-bibliography-of-literature-on-the-rhetoric-of-health-and-medicine/3/

Edwell, J. (2017). Medical interiors: Materiality and spatiality in medical rhetoric. In L. Melonçon & J. B. Scott (Eds.), *Methodologies for the rhetoric of health & medicine* (pp. 157–175). Routledge.

Fang, Y., Li, Z., Chen, H., Zhang, T., Yin, X., Man, J., Yang, X., & Lu, M. (2022). Burden of lung cancer along with attributable risk factors in China from 1990 to 2019, and projections until 2030. *Journal of Cancer Research and Clinical Oncology*. https://doi.org/10.1007/s00432-022-04217-5

Fassin, D. (2018). *Life: A critical user's manual*. Polity Press.

Gouge, C. (2018). Health humanities baccalaureate programs and the rhetoric of health and medicine. *Technical Communication Quarterly*, 27(1), 21–32. https://doi.org/10.1080/10572252.2017.1402566

28   *Toward a theory of patient epistemologies*

Graham, S. S., Kessler, M. M., Kim, S.-Y., Ahn, S., & Card, D. (2018). Assessing perspectivalism in patient participation: An evaluation of FDA patient and consumer representative programs. *Rhetoric of Health & Medicine, 1*(1–2), 58–89. https://doi.org/10.5744/rhm.2018.1006

Hannah, M., & Arduser, L. (2018). Mapping the terrain: Examining the conditions for alignment between the rhetoric of health and medicine and the medical humanities. *Technical Communication Quarterly, 27*(1), 33–49. https://doi.org/10.1080/10572252.2017.1402561

Harper, K. (2020). *The ethos of Black motherhood in America: Only white women get pregnant*. Lexington Books.

Hite, A. H., & Carter, A. (2019). Examining assumptions in science-based policy: Critical health communication, stasis theory, and public health nutrition guidance. *Rhetoric of Health & Medicine, 2*(2), 147–175. https://doi.org/10.5744/rhm.2019.1009

Holladay, D. (2017). Classified conversations: Psychiatry and tactical technical communication in online spaces. *Technical Communication Quarterly, 26*(1), 8–24. https://doi.org/10.1080/10572252.2016.1257744

Joyner, V., Harper, K. C., & Novotny, M. (2023). Introduction to in living color: Amplifying racial justice work in RHM. *Rhetoric of Health & Medicine, 6*(2), 125–142. https://doi.org/10.5744/rhm.2023.6006

Kessler, M. M. (2020). The ostomy multiple: Toward a theory of rhetorical enactments. *Rhetoric of Health & Medicine, 3*(3), 293–319. https://doi.org/10.5744/rhm.2020.1016

Kuehl, R. A., Anderson, J., Drury, S. A. M., Holman, A., Hunt, C., & Leighter, J. L. (2020). Creating a multidisciplinary dialogue about community-based participatory research partnerships of health and medicine. *Rhetoric of Health & Medicine, 3*(1), 93–132. https://doi.org/10.5744/rhm.2020.1004

Larson, S. (2021). *What it feels like: Visceral rhetoric and the politics of rape culture*. PSU Press.

Longtin, K., & Binion, K. (2021). Creating choice and building consensus: Invitational rhetoric as a strategy to promote vasectomies in the United States. *Rhetoric of Health & Medicine, 4*(3), 367–387. https://doi.org/10.5744/rhm.3005

Lynch, J. A., & Zoller, H. (2015). Recognizing differences and commonalities: The rhetoric of health and medicine and critical-interpretive health communication. *Communication Quarterly, 63*(5), 498–503. https://doi.org/10.1080/01463373.2015.1103592

Melonçon, L., & Frost, E. (2015). Special issue introduction: Charting an emerging field: The rhetorics of health and medicine and its importance in communication design. *Communication Design Quarterly, 3*(4), 7–14. https://doi.org/10.1145/2826972.2826973

Melonçon, L., & Scott, J. B. (2017). *Methodologies for the rhetoric of health & medicine*. Taylor & Francis.

Melonçon, L., & Scott, J. B. (2018). Manifesting a scholarly dwelling place in RHM. *Rhetoric of Health & Medicine, 1*(1–2), i–x. https://doi.org/10.5744/rhm.2018.1001

Molloy, C., Beemer, C., Bennett, J., Green, A., Johnson, J., Kessler, M., Novotny, M., & Siegel-Finer, B. (2018). A dialogue on possibilities for embodied methodologies in the rhetoric of health & medicine. *Rhetoric of Health & Medicine, 1*(3–4), 349–371. https://doi.org/10.5744/rhm.2018.1017

Molloy, C., & Hensley Owens, K. (2022). Variants and/in/of the rhetoric of health and medicine. *Rhetoric of Health & Medicine, 5*(1), 1–10. https://doi.org/10.5744/rhm.2022.5001

Novotny, M., & Hertogh, L. B. D. (2022). Amplifying rhetorics of reproductive justice within rhetorics of health and medicine. *Rhetoric of Health & Medicine, 5*(4), 374–402. https://doi.org/10.5744/rhm.2022.5020

Novotny, M., Hertogh, L. B. D., & Frost, E. (2020). Editors' introduction: Rhetorics of reproductive justice in public and civic contexts. *Reflections, 20*(2), 7–14. https://reflectionsjournal.net/wp-content/uploads/2020/12/V20.N2.NovotnyDeHertoghFrost.pdf

Pender, K. (2018). *Being at genetic risk: Toward a rhetoric of care*. PSU Press.

Presley, R. (2021). Kincentricity and Indigenous wellbeing: Food(ways) and/as holistic health in the Native medicine wheel. *Rhetoric of Health & Medicine, 4*(2), 126–157. https://doi.org/10.5744/rhm.2021.2022

Reed, A. (2018). Building on bibliography: Toward useful categorization of research in rhetorics of health and medicine. *Journal of Technical Writing and Communication, 48*(2), 175–198. https://doi.org/10.1177/0047281616667904

Ryan, C. (2021). Exercising uncertainty: Identifying and addressing "grey areas" in a case study involving corporate-funded research on the effects of sugar-sweetened beverages. *Rhetoric of Health & Medicine, 4*(4). https://doi.org/10.5744/rhm.2021.4e3

Sánchez, F. (2020). Distributed and mediated ethos in a mental health call center. *Rhetoric of Health & Medicine, 3*(2), 133–162. https://doi.org/10.5744/rhm.2020.1009

Sastry, S., Zoller, H. M., & Basu, A. (2021). Editorial: Doing critical health communication: A forum on methods. *Frontiers in Communication, 5*. https://doi.org/10.3389/fcomm.2020.637579

Scott, J. B., Molloy, C., & Melonçon, L. (2021). Examining evidence in RHM. *Rhetoric of Health & Medicine, 4*(3), 275–287. https://doi.org/10.5744/rhm.3009

Scott, J. B., Segal, J. Z., & Keranen, L. (2013). The rhetorics of health and medicine: Inventional possibilities for scholarship and engaged practice. *Poroi, 9*(1). https://doi.org/10.13008/2151-2957.1157

Swacha, K., & St Amant, K. (2021). Lego™ learning: A scalable approach to pedagogy in the rhetoric of health and medicine. *Rhetoric of Health & Medicine, 4*(4), 446–474. https://doi.org/10.5744/rhm.4003

Tetteh, J. K., Frimpong, J. B., Budu, E., Adu, C., Mohammed, A., Ahinkorah, B. O., & Seidu, A.-A. (2022). Comprehensive HIV/AIDS knowledge and HIV testing among men in sub-Saharan Africa: A multilevel modelling. *Journal of Biosocial Science, 54*(6), 975–990. https://doi.org/10.1017/S0021932021000560

U.S. Department of Health and Human Services (n.d.). *Social Determinants of Health*. https://health.gov/healthypeople/priority-areas/social-determinants-health

Welhausen, C. A. (2015). Power and authority in disease maps: Visualizing medical cartography through yellow fever mapping. *Journal of Business and Technical Communication, 29*(3), 257–283. https://doi.org/10.1177/1050651915573942

Welhausen, C. A., & Bivens, K. M. (2022). Civilian first responder mHealth apps, interface rhetoric, and amplified precarity. *Rhetoric of Health & Medicine, 5*(1), 11–37. https://doi.org/10.5744/rhm.2022.5002

3 Searching for meaning and support

What women with breast cancer say

When Bryna was diagnosed with cancer for the second time, she joked to Cathryn and Jamie that she once again needed to get a binder to house all the handouts, pamphlets, flyers, and other written artifacts she knew she'd quickly begin to receive from various care providers. Readers who've been diagnosed with an illness, particularly when chronic, can likely relate to the feeling of overwhelm that Bryna was experiencing as she was plunged into a new rhetorical community—the discourses surrounding those with recurrent breast cancer. The materials patients receive from doctors, support groups, and even from loved ones, while intended to inform and support the patient, can have a variety of affective consequences, among them a profound shift in patients' subjectivities. These effects, of course, are often unintended by the author/creator of the document, yet the rhetorical force with which they enter into the scene is undeniable.

To illustrate the cycle of patient epistemologies as we have begun to describe it, this chapter presents the results of a survey and focus groups of women who have undergone treatment for breast cancer. Their participation in our study helped us articulate the iterative process of patient epistemologies by investigating the questions: what discourses do patients encounter and from whom? How do patients interact with these materials and messages in order to make meaning from their illness? We also wanted to know more about the forms of support that were most responsive to patients' needs as they attempted to perform the requisite rhetorical work a person must who: has a cancer diagnosis, is in the midst of cancer treatment(s), has survived cancer and now navigates the chronic physical and mental consequences of various cancer treatments. We asked: what forms of support (e.g., information, actions, others) foster this vital rhetorical work? As this chapter will show, our participants gave us insight into breast cancer patients' perspectives about and experiences with understanding their situation and how forms of information and support played a role in that understanding. In particular, we learned about women's meaning-making in terms of three themes that we elucidate below: making meaning of their situation (absurdity), making meaning about themselves (luck), and taking in information from others (anti-support).

DOI: 10.4324/9781003398318-3

Critiques of breast cancer discourse

There are of course hundreds if not thousands of published studies of clinical breast cancer research, as well as memoirs and narratives that express women's experiences. When we narrow the field to a focus on breast cancer discourse, we encounter studies that analyze women's breast cancer narratives through lenses such as rhetoric, literary or narrative theory, feminism, politics, or other frameworks in disciplines like communications, linguistics, and disabilities studies. For our purposes, we have narrowed our review even further to *critiques* of discourses of cancer, rather than those that establish its features.

Perhaps the two most familiar critiques of breast cancer discourse are Susan Sontag's (1997) *Illness as Metaphor* and Barbara Ehrenreich's (2001) "Welcome to Cancerland." Both are cited prolifically in scholarship on breast cancer. Sontag points out "that the most truthful way of regarding illness – and the healthiest way of being ill – is the one most purified of, most resistant to, metaphoric thinking" (p. 3). And, Ehrenreich calls out discourses that focus on a pink "'marketplace' of breast-cancer-related products to buy" and phony positivity that is anti-feminist and too normalizing of a disease that no one should accept as normal (p. 45). Between the products, the narratives, the ribbons, the walks and fun runs, and the testimonials, Ehrenreich explained:

> "Culture" is too weak a word to describe all this. What has grown up around breast cancer in just the last fifteen years more nearly resembles a cult – or, given that it numbers more than two million women, their families, and friends – perhaps we should say a full-fledged religion.
>
> (p. 50)

Almost all of the research performed on breast cancer culture and discourse references either or both Sontag and Ehrenreich, which is why we also begin with them to review this literature.

Another important and oft-cited study of breast cancer culture and discourse is Maren Klawiter's (2008) *The Biopolitics of Breast Cancer: Changing Cultures of Disease and Activism*. Klawiter is one of the first to trace in depth how breast cancer discourse came to be so pervasive in American culture. In her analysis of the Bay Area breast cancer movement of the 1990s, Klawiter identifies three Cultures of Action (COAs)—culture of early detection and screening activism; culture of patient empowerment and feminist treatment activism; and culture of cancer prevention and environmental activism (p. xxix). Klawiter's cultures are what we would call "rhetorical communities." Each culture, according to Klawiter, is categorized by a common emotion that drives it: hope, anger, and anger, respectively, and each privileges its own discourses of disease (p. xxviii).

Rhetorical scholarship, particularly that found in communication journals, looks at how breast cancer patients are created as discursive subjects in various forms of media. For instance, Tasha Dubriwny (2009) studies how the media coverage surrounding Betty Ford's mastectomy in 1974 solidified femininity as the breast cancer aesthetic, one that still exists 50 years later. Cynthia Ryan (2005) analyzes MAMM magazine, uncovering several ways the magazine counters misleading breast cancer narratives: it uses language about risk rather than "cure;" it presents multiple sides of an issue, allowing readers to decide for themselves; and it doesn't portray breast cancer as a single disease. Karen Kopelson (2013) analyzes the websites for Breast Cancer Action and Breast Cancer Foundation, explaining how these organizations appeal to women using narratives of hope, empowerment, and appeals used by the Komen organization to sell and "recruit to their cause by appealing directly to uncertainty, fear, even chaos" (p. 111).

Critiques of dominant ways of understanding cancer and how they came to be are at the heart of this study. Because Bryna's experiences have not borne out the standard breast cancer narrative, and because we all observed the roteness of the pink ribbons and the gaps in support that Bryna needed, we were particularly inspired by Judy Z. Segal's explanation of agnotology, or the reproduction of cultural ignorance through stagnated discourses—in this case, the standard "survivor" breast cancer narrative. Segal (2008) points out that breast cancer narratives can very often be agnotological, meaning the "standard story of the breast cancer survivor" is to engage in "the cultural production of ignorance" (p. 2). Segal summarizes the standard story: A woman finds a lump in her breast, goes through a series of "battles" to "fight" the cancer (p. 4), and employs this military metaphor so naturally and in a way that it is so entrenched that it is, as Segal says, "not a metaphor at all" (p. 2). The story is always happy, in some ways perhaps even comedic, because we know the narrator has lived to tell it no matter how sad it might get at parts (p. 4). And the closure is that if the reader is like the narrator—if she faces the adversity bravely, transforms terror into triumph, and tells her story—then she will survive and be able to inspire others.

Segal isn't criticizing this standard narrative or the women who write it, but she does want to demonstrate how this entrenched standard makes it nearly impossible to speak about breast cancer in any other way, and therefore, the larger dialogue about breast cancer is never really advanced (p. 18). Segal has suggested that by interrogating agnotological narratives, we can "reinvigorate the conversation" (p. 18). We have sought in this study to interrogate the ways that women make meaning beyond standard narratives, and even beyond narrative itself. In doing so, we asked our research participants *not* to tell their stories, but to tell us the *other* rhetorical forms that comprised their breast cancer experience, as the results section below will explain. This emphasis on *what else*, rhetorically speaking, is available to women at health flashpoints, also bears out in Chapters 4 and 5 on menopause and sobriety respectively.

Methodology and methods

Methodological approach

As noted in the introduction, we use a variation on a multiple ontological vantage as a methodological orientation to patients' experiences to show which sources of information might be useful and which forms of support helpful, as well as to highlight something arguably more ineffable and difficult to trace: how, in day-to-day rhetorical practice, these things become integral, everyday parts of a person's attempts to live a good life in the context of frightening diagnoses, grueling treatment regimes, and uncertain potential futures. These ineffable and difficult-to-trace rhetorical practices, we contend, constitute an episteme. We wanted to know more about the variety of sources of information that helped patients to make sense of what they were going through and about the sources of information that helped them to make difficult decisions related to their care and their lives. Our work, then, relies on Mol's who, in invoking care, "wants us to focus on what it is that patients do in order to live a good life when what they really want—perfect health—is not possible" (Pender, 2018, p. 21). As such, we asked women to tell us what was most helpful and supportive to them in their breast cancer diagnosis, treatment, and aftercare because we think these are crucial components to the profound rhetorical work that leads to new knowledge. Our inquiry went in a different, more granular, and less concrete direction than a study of patient education materials that looks at such issues as legibility or usability might.

Participant recruitment

This portion of our study began with survey research that included both quantitative and qualitative measures (see https://patientsmakingmeaning.com/ for survey questionnaire). This survey was fully anonymous, yet it ended with an invitation to link to a second, non-anonymous survey where participants could indicate their willingness to participate in a focus group. We were fortunate enough to be granted approval to access the ABOUT Network participant membership (ABOUT is not an acronym). Self-described as a "patient-powered network," the ABOUT Network is a research registry that was created by Facing Our Risk of Cancer Empowered (FORCE) in collaboration with researchers from the University of South Florida (aboutnetwork.org). The data registry contains information from 10,500 men and women who have voluntarily taken a survey to share their cancer experiences. The ABOUT Network advertised and recruited participants for our study through email blasts and via social media posts that were targeted to our participant criterion: any person over the age of eighteen who has ever been diagnosed with breast cancer.

We also recruited participants using this same criterion by posting links to our survey on our own social media accounts where we asked those in our networks to consider participating and to share the opportunity with their networks, and, thus, making use of snowball sampling. Fifty-one people completed surveys, and eight women joined our focus groups—Kayla, Leslie, Lauren, Melissa, Sally, Leah, Karina, and Martha (pseudonyms). In the focus groups, we used questions as listed on our website (https://patientsmakingmeaning.com/).

Given the relatively small number of study participants, we see this data as a starting point in making sense of the cycle of patient epistemologies. While we do not see it as an indication of what happens with all patients with breast cancer, the study serves as an illustration of how information and support are variously deployed, understood, and used (or not) in the complex rhetorical work of making sense of a health flashpoint and of rehearsing, performing, and redoing everyday decision-making in light of this rhetorical work. Our contribution, thus, is a theoretical one; this chapter builds theory that is intentionally adaptable. The theoretical construct it puts forward can and should be reshaped, challenged, and repurposed with and for a wide variety of human beings across the globe experiencing a range of health flashpoints.

Procedures

Surveys were conducted via an anonymous Qualtrics link, and focus groups took place over Zoom in December 2020. We chose to do survey research because we wanted to capture sensitive demographic data on participants while also getting more information on the sources of information and forms of support that helped or hindered their rhetorical work and decision-making related to their cancer experiences. We also held focus groups in order to gain more information on how participants used information and support as they made new knowledge for themselves related to their breast cancer experiences.

While we reasoned that interviews could provide depth of understanding, we also were aware that participants would be asked to talk through highly affect-inducing health experiences. From surveys, we learned that breast cancer patients strongly prefer to gain information from others who have had breast cancer. We thus reasoned that focus groups would foster environments in which participants could have a conversation with others who have also had breast cancer rather than talking one-on-one with a researcher who may or may not have had cancer. While we do not claim to have obtained perfect data, we honor participants' labor, openness, and candor in using it to build a theory of patient epistemology that could be productively used and adapted in future study.

Coding

Our data analysis began with the first cycle coding method of "structural coding" wherein we both coded and initially categorized "the data corpus to examine comparable segments' commonalities, differences, and relationships" (Saldaña, 2021, p. 130). Such that we could apply a "content-based or conceptual phrase representing a topic of inquiry to a larger segment of the data" (Saldaña, 2021, p. 130), we identified what sources of information and forms of support were apparent in the data we had. We then used pattern coding to further drill down into our data; two researchers read each transcript and open-ended survey responses. We next met to reconcile and solidify our code book, and a third researcher read each of the transcripts and survey responses to code using this code book, which is shown with examples in Table 3.1.

After second stage coding was completed, we met once again to discuss the data and our findings, leading us to develop the cycle of patient epistemologies described in Chapter 1—health flashpoint leads to affective response, which then leads to rhetorical work, to material and constitutive effects, and to reflection, and back and forth, or again.

As Chapter 2 makes clear, patient epistemologies unfold as health flashpoints, giving way to affective jolts that shift patient subjectivities and propel them into purposeful rhetorical work meant to aid crucial, day-to-day decision-making. With these terms in mind, we arranged our coded data into key themes for discussion and reportage: 1) absurdity; 2) luck; and 3) anti-support. Our codes variously enter into these three themes, yet these themes allow us to do the theory-building we wish to do in a way that marching through an explanation of our codes with examples would not have done. Below, we explicate each of these themes and discuss how our data led us to them as well as how they allow us to put forward a theory of patient epistemologies.

Discussion/results

Absurdity

When we looked to our data to help us conceptualize how patients make meaning from sources of information and forms of support, we arrived at a surprising insight: absurdity plays a major role in the ways that patients report having conceptualized and made meaning of their experiences. We define "absurd" in line with the Oxford English Dictionary (2021): "against or without reason or propriety; incongruous, unreasonable, illogical; acting in an incongruous, unreasonable, or illogical manner." Absurdity invokes that which has no place and is out of place. Likewise, we see these ways of making meaning as wrapped up in the rhetorical concept of *aporia* that account for the internal contradiction, the logical disjunction that participants shared: how a person is extrapolated from life as they knew it into a conceptual set of contradictions that leave them nowhere yet carries some epistemological weight.

Absurdity plays out in the data in two major ways that are not necessarily distinct: (1) that time and life "go on" while a person experiences breast cancer and (2) a rift in expectations occurs around the timeline of one's illness,

Table 3.1 Code Book

Code	Definition	Example
Aporia/ absurdity	Ways that participants' situations seemed illogical yet possibly amusing or ironic	"I was super lucky that a colleague of mine was diagnosed with the same sort of breast cancer."
Anti-support	Ways that others failed at supporting the participant or caused the participant to feel the opposite of supported	"People would always offer food. And there was always that sort of element of insult when we would say, no, we don't want that."
Cancer	Specific discussion of illness or treatment	"You know, I had a lump after the breast cancer."
Decision-making	Expressions of doubt, lack of information, making a decision about treatment or care	"So I think for me personally, making a decision about whether or not to keep your breasts, I think, you know, your partner is going to be intimately involved in that decision."
Doctor-provided documents	Brochures, pamphlets, others provided by medical practitioners; usefulness of these materials	"They sent me home with, like, a folder, full of pamphlets, which I don't think I read a single one."
Informational needs/ preferences	Conducting research, going "down a rabbit hole," usefulness and specificity of materials	"If I feel like I'm not getting the information that I want, I might go look for it."
Luck	Referring to gratitude or being/feeling lucky in the context of illness, comparing experience to others	"And then you know you're surrounded by like women who, like, have it much harder, much more challenging journeys, and you realize like, you know, you really did get lucky."
Material support	Non-text support; support such as meals, cards, etc.	"I had friends and colleagues who organized a meal train… and it wasn't just meals for me and my family, but also little cards and little things for my daughter, who was younger at the time."
Need for resources	Descriptions of the types of resources needed during treatment, such as childcare, insurance approval, certain information	"And so they called the social worker and she arrived and I probably didn't need help with the insurance paper, but the—well I know I didn't—but the word 'help' sounded good."

(Continued)

Table 3.1 (Continued)

Code	Definition	Example
Patient education background	Discussion of the participant's own education, level of understanding complex medical information	"Somewhat of a respect of my own life in academia, my ability as a researcher to read materials, and I think that provided for a different level of support."
People/ support	Describing a particular person and how they supported the participant, identifying a particular person or group as having been supportive	"I feel like I probably identify more with my breast cancer surgeon, she's a similar age, you know, we have kids that are similar age. So I probably identified more with her."
Performing sickness/ external perceptions of illness	Ways participants felt like they had to show to others that they were sick; feeling as if they are not believed unless they demonstrate sickness	"People often told me how great I looked- I thought this was nice but somewhat odd how often people said it to me. I almost thought- am I supposed to look like a corpse or something?"
Race	Referring to race	"As a Black person, as a Black woman, I've had plenty of negative, like mildly negative... doesn't have to be really like severe for it to be a negative experience. Um, you know, it could be pretty what you might call minor micro-aggression..."
Rhetorical analysis	Performing analysis of documents provided by the researchers or other documents	"I scoured the internet for information, but I, very much aware of how dangerous the internet can be and how there's a ton of really bad information out there. So I scoured the internet, but I was also very careful about the sources that I chose and I probably read a dozen articles on this, on this website and a couple other, you know, more reputable websites."
Time	Referring to passage of time	"Yeah, life carries on. Right, like there's other, other things in life besides breast cancer."
Writing	Talking about their own writing, blogging, or other kind of text production.	"I also began my own blog on caringbridge.org which was helpful to me to share my information with others."

with patients experiencing cancer as acute and chronic simultaneously. As Bryna put it to Jamie and Cathryn, this category could be summed up with "My life was still a thing that I was doing, and I was also doing cancer. But doing both together influenced how I did cancer and how I did my life." Thinking of absurdity and aporia help us to articulate how participants have had to navigate their cancer diagnosis, treatment, and aftercare as acute and chronic at the same time. For example, as one participant put it, "Yeah, life carries on. Right, like there's other, other things in life besides breast cancer."

Our participants revealed that they felt expected to (and indeed did) live in the material conditions of aporia: namely, they are ill, yet they must carry on with business as usual while simultaneously "doing" illness and all that it entails. They must keep up with chemotherapies, for instance, and make decisions on and possibly undergo surgical procedures, but they must also make sure the car gets inspected, the kids get to school, and the unsafe tree gets removed. In all cases, the mundane tasks and special occasions of everyday life were still present as if the world had not shifted, so the patient must live both in their previous reality as if it were not layered over with a completely different and contradictory new reality that not everyone else knows about, sees, or acknowledges and of which children certainly are not fully aware.

Relatedly, for the women in our study, the health flashpoint of a cancer diagnosis meant that time itself took on a contradictory quality. Swept up into a health flashpoint, the person gets diagnosed, and within minutes, they are getting a course of treatment without time or space to say what they want, need, prefer, what their options are, and/or where there are resources to attend to very specific needs. They must press on with this new life and contend with the fact that their "old" daily life is still happening. Many participants expressed ways that they were mourning expectations for a planned biographical life—as they attempted to build careers and parent young children, for example. As Leslie explained:

> Life is busy, I was busy. I mean, that's true for everyone, I wasn't unique or special in that way at all. But when I got the cancer diagnosis, but it was like, well, this is a really bad time. I've got this and this and this and this and this. You want me to have surgery and like right, right away and then chemotherapy. Well, what the heck? Anyway, so it was like, I'm only going to do what's going to work and what's not going to take my energy away from me.

In this case, cancer treatments taking over her entire life and depleting all of her time and energy seemed like it could not be an appropriate option, yet the course of treatment meant that Leslie's "real" life would inevitably take a background role while cancer treatments took center stage. In the end, as we mentioned in Chapter 2, Leslie did indeed put her "real" life first, making the decision to delay treatment until an important family milestone could happen:

I was going to delay chemotherapy till after my daughter's birthday. I thought that was a brilliant plan; the oncologist disagreed, but I think if the healthcare community could understand that you really can't treat a parent without providing them support for their kids, because, right, most parents will walk into a train for their kid, right? Like it's not and I, how, how can a person focus on treatment and getting well if their child's not taken care of.

In this and other remarks, we detected that forms of support or sources of information that did not take partners and especially children's needs into account felt flat and impeded a productive cycle of patient epistemologies.

A form of absurdity that also appeared in our data was centered around the concepts of acute and chronic illness timelines. Women expressed that they had been given information that indicated to them that their cancer experiences would end once they completed treatment, suggesting that the acute emergency of cancer would at some point come to an end. However, many described a series of chronic mental and physical health consequences that resulted in a need to continue the cycle of patient epistemologies indefinitely. Martha explained:

It is such a mental game when you are done. I was so much more depressed and withdrawn when it was all over. It takes a lot to find a new norm and accept that you will always have this fear of cancer returning in the back of your mind and your body never feels the same.

Similarly, Melissa told us:

After the big dismissal where you get to ring the bell, and, and leave and stuff and you know at that point, you're so reliant on those people. It's like you're leaving your family and friends, but they give you a bunch of stuff to take with you. And at that point, then I was really ready to dive into some things and so I would know what was going to come next [even after treatment and being "done"].

Notably, Melissa was very aware that she was ready to turn to the support she'd received for aftercare and she moved into the reflection part of the epistemological process with purpose.

Luck

A sizable part of the agnotological narrative of breast cancer (Segal, 2008) is the undercurrent that characterizes so many interactions that participants engaged in: the minute you experience the health flashpoint of a breast cancer diagnosis, you are always, quite simply, characterized as lucky that you're still alive. The implication is that a person should be happy they've been diagnosed and eager for treatment—a stale and agnotological narrative that precludes thinking or change in attitudes. Luck, imbued as it has become in the standard narrative, did indeed show up in our data seemingly because we are all steeped in this narrative, with participants describing their luck relative to the alternative—a cancer experience that ends in death. We see this as also invoking aporia as, of course, what would be thought of as "lucky" when the alternative is death is not necessarily lucky at all; true luck would be never having had cancer to begin with, yet that reality has been entirely foreclosed upon once a patient is ushered into the rhetorical community of breast cancer.

As our participant Sally put it, "luckily, so far, my diagnosis was quite a while ago," meaning that she considers her situation one of good fortune because she has not had a recurrence. It's very likely that Sally picked up this idea from the various forms of rhetorical work that have characterized her own ways of making meaning out of her breast cancer experiences. As Karina similarly stated:

> The sort of breast cancer that I had was, you know, sort of like the lucky one to get which [she felt bitter about because] you know, the breast cancer surgeon who said that to me at the time…did not have the experience to know that that is true.

In this case, Karina got the message that she should begin to conceptualize herself as among the lucky because hers was not as aggressive as other forms of cancer. A survey respondent articulated this viewpoint as well when they wrote, "I was lucky that my appearance didn't change much, which probably helped more than I can truly understand." This participant felt lucky, then, that she didn't have to see a sick person in the mirror and, thus, did not have to confront the full weight of this new subjectivity. Other women, such as Martha, felt lucky to have good support: "So I lucked out in that way and my family, my family was pretty good, too." Perhaps the "feel lucky" imperative does some good in terms of patient epistemologies as it could lead to positive thinking with some benefits.

We suggest that the persistent assumption that a cancer diagnosis that is not an imminent death sentence is lucky seems to lead to these other declarations of luck; we suspect that the idea of luck might also undermine the possibility of epistemology that these experiences bring with them. This narrative of luck, pervasive in discourses surrounding cancers that do not swiftly kill the patient, can lead to patients feeling unsupported or even offended. As Martha put it:

> The only time I felt a bit offended was when someone close to me told me I was lucky. No doubt, I had an easier treatment, prognosis, and path than many. Yes, I was so lucky, and I still am; but until you go through treatments you really should not make that statement.

In this case, the participant does not feel so lucky after all, so when forms of support or sources of information hinge on this idea that if you are not dead or going to be soon, that qualifies as "luck," there can be unintended consequences. Additionally, luck, as an aporetic device, can forestall important affective responses and hence epistemological work. Drawbacks in the trope of the lucky-because-not-deadly cancer narrative are worth further attention.

Anti-support

Something we found most surprising in our data was the role that what we call "anti-support" plays in the cycle of patient epistemologies. We define "anti-support" as those attempts by friends, family members, care providers, and casual acquaintances to provide sources of information and/or forms of support that are clearly intended to have ameliorative effects, yet these attempts do not end up being all that supportive after all for a variety of reasons. We suggest that anti-support disrupts and impedes or unintentionally alters a productive recursive cycle of patient epistemologies as they place additional mental, emotional, and intellectual burdens on patients when, as our section on absurdity makes clear, they are already operating in incongruent temporalities.

The upshot of this evidence is that it is some of the first researched evidence of how breast cancer patients honestly reacted and think about very common forms of "support" such as meal trains. Below, we offer them in a practical sense, a sort of "Do/Do Not" list that shows how people, in choosing commonly understood help actions without critical thought to a process of epistemology which will be unique to each patient, not only ignore that the well-intended person's actions are contributing to the person's meaning-making but in some cases, actively work to produce a more confounded, absurd, and potentially bitter experience. The irony is that attitudes and platitudes that come from a place of neatness and closure—despite common perceptions of narrative being a main way to help people work through many types of life challenges—actually work toward disrupting the kind of experience that friends and family might be wishing for the patient and work more toward making their absurd sick/well life more socially and emotionally fraught and difficult for them.

For example, as Kayla explained:

> My wife's colleagues took up a collection to get us meals sent pretty regularly and also to have somebody come clean our house. So this is like the positive and the negative at the same time. So, my wife was adamantly opposed to allowing a stranger to come in and clean our house. So this was like the super generous gift and I was like, "hell yeah" but she was not having it so, so she had to very delicately tell her closest coworker that we couldn't use that part of the gift.

The sentiment behind supporting a colleague's cancer treatment experiences with a cleaning service to take the burden of household chores off the family's to-do list was, as Kayla knew, a very nice one. However, it turned to anti-support when the burden of declining the gift fell on the family, thus adding to their burden rather than lightening it.

Similarly, food gifts—universally acknowledged as kind to give—can tend toward anti-support. As Lauren explained:

> There was that tendency of people who, especially since we're in the Midwest, that it's like, how do you help people? You bring food. Um, and there was a real, real insistence that, um, we had to accept the food that people were offering. Now, one thing that was actually happening was, um, my treatment really wasn't that bad. And I was, um, you know, especially after what she had gone through, um, and genuinely cooking or things like that were like, okay. And in fact ways to, um, interact particularly with my younger daughter, but people would always offer food. And there was always that sort of element of insult when we would say, no, we don't want that.

For Lauren, food preparation was something she could do and enjoyed doing, a daily task that during her illness actually functioned as a touchstone to the everyday life that she was attempting to maintain. For her, preparing food was a way to stay connected to her daughter and a way for her to feel normal. Rather than feeling supported by others' insistence on bringing food, she felt burdened by both having to refuse the offers and by having to deal with the inevitable hurt feelings when she did decline the food offers.

Lauren also articulated the ways that anti-support played a role in her experiences with breast cancer diagnosis, treatment, and aftercare. As she noted:

> Um, but in the support group, we used to joke about it in terms of like, people feel they have to do something, so they do something and then they kind of go, like, I [the well-intended person] feel better now. Without that sense of, um, you know, I was really concerned about making *you* feel better about this. A lot of people were understanding about it, but a lot of people would be like almost insulted when we said, you know, food's not really what we need right now.

Other participants found aphorisms that have become cancer tropes to be highly problematic forms of anti-support. Lauren explained:

> I know, like, you know, have been to the cancer experience with his patients and his family members, um, do often joke about the God only gives you all that you can handle, um, statement. That seems to be one

that people love to say. And one that people hate to hear, um, because it's, um, you know, it just has, it's very problematic and along the same lines, occasionally, um, people will, um, talk about 'Thank God my family is healthy' to you. Or, you know, 'I very nearly was diagnosed with breast cancer too.' It's like, okay, um, this is not so much about you, you know, that kind of thing, but, but those kinds of platitudes.

Platitudes are not always the helpful reminders that they are likely meant to be—a declaration of the patients' strength and resilience, a reminder, perhaps, that a higher being is looking out for or even rooting for the patient to make a full recovery. However, patients hear these things as forms of dismissal, as invalidators of suffering, and as indictments against reasonable fear and worry over prognosis.

Similarly, another form of anti-support also involved individuals centering themselves rather than the person experiencing cancer. A survey respondent wrote:

> Numerous people had an emotional response when I told them I'd been diagnosed with cancer. It brought up their experiences with someone they loved who'd had cancer. Some people cried. I often ended up comforting them. While I understand how hard it is to watch someone you love go through cancer treatment, I didn't have the energy to comfort them and take care of myself.

Patients also found anecdotal experiences to be forms of anti-support, such as Sally, who told us about the people in her life who'd suggested that they could understand her cancer experiences because of a third party's experiences, "Oh my, you know, my friend had breast cancer. And this is what she did. So this is what you should do. You know, you get like a lot of the armchair doctors." Karina similarly expressed, "I was annoyed by a few in the support group who were know-it-alls and always had something to say even when their journey didn't involve chemo or if they didn't like a surgeon that others loved." A survey participant had a similar remark:

> I was annoyed with people who would tell me about a friend or family member that died from cancer or that I should try juicing, becoming vegan, or doing only holistic treatments as they perceived chemo to "kill." I was also annoyed with people who would tell me that I got a "free boob job" and didn't understand the severity of the surgery or my cancer. I would get annoyed with a family member who left the clinical nursing field 25 years ago but would insist that I listen to her instead of the advice of my oncologist. I get annoyed with the unsolicited advice.

For this survey participant, it is very clear that a productive epistemological cycle is thwarted by well-intended people doing and saying wrong and hurtful things. Another survey participant had a similar experience:

> The most hurtful comments for someone with incurable cancer are those where people think they know what you are going through or compare your situation to one of their own that does not come close to comparing. Also when others try to tell you what to do to get cured when there is no cure out there. Sometimes it is difficult when well-meaning people think that they know what is best for you medically when they have no idea.

Clearly, comparing a person's cancer experience to other people's experiences and to dissimilar cases does damage and is not at all supportive.

Participants also found the tendency for their experiences to be "pink-washed" or swept up into the breast cancer industrial complex as well as references to bravery and to survivorship to be forms of anti-support. As one participant put it:

> Telling me I'm brave gets on my nerves or that I'm so strong. My definition of brave isn't about cancer, it's about those that put their life on the line daily. They have the choice to do that, whereas cancer didn't give me the choice. I either do the treatment and hope for the best or die.

Another participant echoed this same concern, explaining, "like survivor is hero sort of idea. Like you had accomplished something great because you survived, you know, like what else were you supposed to do?"

Similarly, another survey respondent explained:

> Unhelpful: But how are you, really? Usually voiced in a mournful cadence & tone. Also unhelpful: I know this pink little bear will make you feel happy which is what you need to survive this. Nope, I only felt better when my treatments were over, when I get a good report and when I watched the little pink bear be driven away by the garbage truck.

Martha summed up experiences with anti-support: "people have their own ideas about, like, what support looks like." Often, the failure of support or anti-support is more about not feeling heard or seen with one's particular experience. In that case, the well-intended people are being affected by social norms or internal feelings of duty rather than simply asking what they can do. It puts a burden on the sick person to say "no" to help that is unwanted or not right for the circumstance. It also perpetuates the agnotological narrative that sick people or people with cancer simply need the same support that all sick people or prior people with cancer in someone's past experience needed. Or, that a helper only has or needs one way of helping (e.g., bringing a lasagna) in any sick-person circumstance. Yet the women we interviewed rebuked this; they want more thoughtful, customized, individualized support that does not rest on selfishness, agnotology, or assumptions.

Conclusion and implications

Our participants shared with us their experiences, emotions, and opinions in honest and raw ways. We observed that the opportunities afforded to the participants by our study to write and talk seemed to constitute an additional opportunity to make meaning, and some of the participants confirmed that— that they are never done thinking, talking, processing, and making new decisions about their health and lives since their cancer diagnosis and treatment. They welcomed the chance to talk with other survivors in this capacity as well. The very act of interacting with our participants in this manner helped us to conceive of the process of epistemologies overall.

Participants' recollections of their experiences made it clear that forms of support that would acknowledge the absurdity of their situation, provide more thoughtful support, and avoid platitudes would also include practical things such as babysitting and rides to treatment, as well as a revision of frames of mind or language use. Instead of neat narrative closure or platitudes, as in forms of support and sources of information that indicate the following arc: "I got diagnosed with cancer, I did cancer treatment, and I got my life back," evidence from our study is strongly in favor of an opposite disposition: the health flashpoint of a cancer diagnosis is one part of a cyclical and meandering experience that must co-occur with "real life" and then, never really ends. Such a reframing makes it more possible that something that many participants said was not enough a consideration would be given its due: the need for continuous follow-up care in the context of chronic consequences of treatment.

The reader will note in this chapter a somewhat negative or critical tone about the ways in which information and support are considered by the participants. We deem this an important contribution to the discourse of breast cancer patient experience, as we offer the assertion that friends, family, and support people are perhaps overly motivated by uncritical assumptions or socially-approved scripts or tropes for supporting women with breast cancer, and that not enough alternatives exist.

We contend that these patients' perspectives and critiques are helpful in shaping alternative ways of supporting patients, and that one of those ways is to consider how one, through language, is *always already* contributing to a patients' epistemological process during illness. Without that awareness, triteness and uncritical unhelpfulness feature prominently in a patient's experience, mostly probably unbeknownst to the well-intended people. With awareness of the themes presented in this chapter, we assert that caretakers and support people can question and perhaps upend their own assumptions and then revise or invent if not new ways of support, then individualized ways that focus on the real-life circumstances of the patient. This will go a ways toward removing extra and unnecessary stressors in their loved one's experience.

The reader might also take away four implications related to patient epistemologies that will bear out in the following chapters as well:

1. meaning-making is a process that can unwittingly be shaped, interrupted, or foreclosed through well-meaning but agnotological discourse surrounding the patient
2. meaning-making is an iterative process, and that with time and reflection, new meanings will emerge and become relevant to one's health over the lifespan
3. women often still don't have the language for what they went through; that they use terms like 'journey,' 'luck,' and 'survivor' with a knowing reluctance for well-understood yet not fully appropriate expressions; that the experience is often characterized by regret, anger, bad memories, and uncaring and uncritical people and comments
4. supporters can and should attend to the meaning-making experience, rather than taking a gamble on contributing to it in an uncritical way.

References

Dubriwny, T. (2009). Constructing breast cancer in the news: Betty Ford and the evolution of the breast cancer patient. *Journal of Communication Inquiry, 33*(2), 104–125. https://doi.org/10.1177/0196859908329090

Ehrenreich, B. (2001, November). Welcome to cancerland: A mammogram leads to a cult of pink kitsch. *Harper's*, 43–53. https://archive.harpers.org/2001/11/pdf/HarpersMagazine-2001-11-0075358.pdf?AWSAccessKeyId=AKIAJUM7PFZHQ4PMJ4LA&Expires=1568333045&Signature=HWjBLPajQSIfCgZFDl1dhshivZc%3D

Klawiter, M. (2008). *The biopolitics of breast cancer: Changing cultures of disease and activism.* University of Minnesota Press.

Kopelson, K. (2013). Risky appeals: Recruiting to the environmental breast cancer movement in the age of "pink fatigue." *Rhetoric Society Quarterly, 43*(2), 107–133. https://doi.org/10.1080/02773945.2013.768350

Oxford English Dictionary Online. (2021). *absurd, adj. 1a.* Oxford University Press. https://www.oed.com/viewdictionaryentry/Entry/792#:~:text=Thesaurus%20%C2%BB-,a.,%3B%20incongruous%2C%20unreasonable%2C%20illogical

Pender, K. (2018). *Being at genetic risk: Toward a rhetoric of care.* Penn State University Press.

Ryan, C. (2005). Struggling to survive: A study of editorial decision-making strategies at MAMM magazine. *Journal of Business and Technical Communication, 19*(3), 353–376. https://doi.org/10.1177/1050651905275643

Saldaña, J. (2021). *The coding manual for qualitative researchers* (4th ed.). SAGE Publications.

Segal, J. Z. (2008). Breast cancer narratives as public rhetoric: Genre itself and the maintenance of ignorance. *Linguistics and the Human Sciences, 3*(1), 3–23. https://doi.org/10.1558/lhs.v3i1.3

Sontag, S. (1977). *Illness as metaphor.* Farrar, Straus and Giroux.

4 Entering the conversation

Rhetorical encounters with a stagnated menopause discourse

As the previous two chapters demonstrate, the making and remaking of patient epistemologies is a continual process wherein a health flashpoint can cause an individual to be thrust into a rhetorical community that was not of their own choosing. Health flashpoints are often characterized by affective responses, yet they also mean that decisions need to be made. This decision-making, we have argued, is bolstered via diverse rhetorical work. Rhetorical work leads to material and constitutive effects, to reflection, to more rhetorical work, to more decision-making, and, quite often, the process continues on as more health flashpoints enter the scene. It has been the thesis of this book thus far that in this frenetic and cyclical energy, new knowledge is constantly being created and recreated as patients navigate everyday life in the context of their health and the potential for medical interventions and various supports that they can opt into or not. This chapter continues this meditation on the cycle of patient epistemologies by focusing on the health flashpoint of menopause or, more precisely, perimenopausal symptoms that eventually lead to the full cessation of menses, or menopause.

We explore this topic via a corpus of recent texts that we gathered by relying on Kristi Cole and Anna Carmon's (2019) adaptation of Han Park's (2003) "observation on a hyperlinked network" (p. 293)—a tactic we explain in detail below. To analyze our corpus and to reach conclusions, we used critical discourse analysis (CDA) via a theoretical orientation to the rhetorical concept of *doxa* or popular opinion as a guiding principle—also explicated further below. Through examining the materials and messages that exist in English for women and those assigned female at birth who are experiencing the health flashpoint of menopause, and by looking at the likely rhetorical encounters related to how to navigate this stage of life, we are able to uncover a notable trend: sources of information about perimenopause and menopause over the decades consistently and repeatedly claim that there is not enough information out there and that there are not enough support structures in place to make this phase of life livable. These texts also claim that the time for silence has ended, and women must demand space to talk about and gain support during this critical time in their lives.

However, a deeper look at this body of work reveals that the claim of "no information out there" repeats over time and through many generations and

DOI: 10.4324/9781003398318-4

iterations. Our analysis in this chapter leads us to argue that this repetition causes stagnation and less attention on how and why perimenopause and menopause are so difficult; we claim that sexism and not insufficient information is to blame. Much like Brenna Matlock's (2021) wherein she demonstrated that too much focus on the novelty of women working in conventional weapons destruction limits deeper engagements with this interesting group of post-conflict workers, we argue that too many texts claiming that lack of information is to blame for menopause being an unpleasant and unsupported phase of life take attention away from the real culprit—misogyny, and especially abject hatred of older and aging women—a well-documented cultural phenomenon that is nonetheless too rarely equated with the difficulties encountered in this health flashpoint (Åberg et al., 2020; Chrisler, 2011; Nosek et al., 2010; Syme & Cohn, 2016). Likewise, we claim that the disagreements that emerge in the bodies of knowledge on whether menopause is a medical disease or a natural process create a definitional crisis that allows the more pressing dimensions of menopause to be deemphasized, flattened, or even erased.

When women begin to experience symptoms of perimenopause and seek out sources of information and forms of support, they are likely to encounter a variety of media that take as a starting point the idea that menopause has not received enough attention. A recent example can be found in a popular *New York Times* piece that says that women have been "misled" about menopause and that too few women know about the true benefit-risk ratio for menopausal hormone therapy (Dominus, 2023). Even articles about menopause that would seem to focus on crucial issues, such as indicating that menopause can be different for women of color, focus on the fact that all women have little-to-no guidance when they begin this phase of life (Gupta, 2023), and other texts focus on how the wellness industry is monetizing menopause (Larocca, 2022).

While these sources make it seem like there is a cultural shift surrounding menopause happening currently, we observe that discourses surrounding menopause, in fact, are stuck in a loop and don't move beyond a few predictable patterns and categories of information that we outline herein. The consequence of this loop is a lack of attention to the real issues women face when they reach this health flashpoint and grapple with attendant affect. When women reach this health flashpoint, in other words, we argue that women might suffer not from a lack of information on what is happening with their bodies, but from the subtle, yet profound effects of the diffuse and indeterminate mix of misogyny and ageism that has been gradually internalized. Still, the dominant message to women at this health flashpoint has remained stagnant: you don't have enough information, and information will empower you to get through this transition and to end the silence about this life stage.

For instance, in Gail Sheehy's (1992) bestseller *The Silent Passage*, she urged women to take charge of their menopause transitions with ideas and themes that permeate myriad texts on this topic over time—that women should end the silence enshrouding this common experience, explore clinical and homeopathic treatments for symptoms, focus on diet and exercise to ease the transition, embrace this "second puberty," and look forward to what could be, with the right preparation, a new and empowering phase of life. A theme in Sheehy's text is that the time of silence around menopause is coming to an end and that women should proactively contribute to their own health liberation by arming themselves with good information and then using that information to advocate for the care that they want and need. With then-modern treatment options, an end to vitality as women age, Sheehy argued, is not a foregone conclusion. While the book was widely read, led to a number of ancillary publications in popular media, and went through several reprints (with the most recent one in 2010), not much appears to have shifted in the discourses surrounding menopause following its successes.

Indeed, various recent, public-facing media we analyze below now, three decades later, argue that women are in desperate need of sources of information and forms of support related to menopause—an experience that remains shrouded in silence, shame, and stigma. Some sources claim, in fact, either directly or tacitly, that we are in the midst of a "menopause renaissance" in which women finally have the opportunity to do exactly what Sheehy said was already well underway in the early 1990s—to once and for all end their silent suffering, to get the information they need, and to seek out the supportive clinical and/or homeopathic therapies and remedies that best fit their own bodies, histories, comfort levels, and desires. And while more recent texts, of course, include insights from more up-to-date health and medical research and treatment options, *the basic arguments, underlying assumptions, and suggestions are remarkably similar*: women who've been in the dark about this experience need to be empowered to take on the menopause transition armed with knowledge and ready to insist on quality care from providers and on compassion and understanding from family, friends, and employers; the silence needs to end. Public interest in menopause, though, hardly started with Sheehy, and her book does make sense as a feminist-lite response to another popular menopause-related text that emerged in the 1960s.

In 1966, Robert Wilson published his popular text *Feminine Forever*, a book that argued that menopause is the medical problem or disease of hormone deficiency and, thus, it can be corrected for the remainder of a woman's life via hormone replacement therapies (HRTs). His wildly misogynist argument was that frustrated husbands could have their wives remain agreeable, pretty, and sexual if they convinced them to take HRTs. As Jen Gunter's (2021) recent book *The Menopause Manifesto* explained, Wilson's (1966) book and related research led to a number of complementary popular publications in a slew of magazines and newspapers where even women who'd not read the book were given that same message—that menopause is a preventable medical disease, and that going through its youth-ravishing unpleasantness could be prevented with a simple, steady course of HRTs.

As Judith A. Houck (2003) explained, women's responses to Wilson's claims were already divided by the time studies linking HRTs to endometrial cancer began to emerge in the mid-1970s with some women embracing the promise of continued vitality and others critiquing the pathologization of women's normal human aging processes, and those studies managed to shift the discourses around menopause without necessarily creating any consensus on what menopause *is* (disease or natural process) and how it should, therefore, be treated (or not). Just as the repetition of the message that menopause is perpetually shrouded in secrecy and ignorance does damage, the lack of consensus on what menopause *is* (a medical condition warranting clinical interventions, a natural phase of life meant to be endured, or something in-between) not only leaves the general public understandably confused, but it also contributes to a stagnation of themes and concepts explored in texts related to menopause; it creates the conditions in which the constant message that there is insufficient information on menopause can be repeated unchecked.

In an attempt to counter the claim that menopause is a disease, Gunter's (2021) book makes a number of intentional moves. For example, Gunter called for women to use the term "menopausal hormone therapy" (MHT) to draw attention to the fact that in post-menopausal women, missing hormones aren't necessarily being replaced, but symptoms are, instead, being addressed using an appropriate therapy that women can carefully choose after weighing personal benefits to risks based on the best available data. In other words, Gunter is clearly of the opinion that menopause is a natural process that can nonetheless benefit from medical intervention. That said, most texts don't stake a clear claim in terms of whether menopause is a disease or a natural process. Most texts, Gunter's included, also operate under the assumption that women are caught in a perpetual state of knowing nothing about, and are, thus, likely to feel totally blindsided by menopause and that they are simultaneously very likely to encounter resistance, denial, and poor quality of care when they bring perimenopausal and post-menopausal concerns to their care providers.

Thus, popular discourses, in this way, respond to the confusion not by finally resolving the definitional crisis surrounding menopause, but by lamenting the silence and stigma surrounding menopause and by giving women lists of symptoms they might expect and a number of mechanisms (from self-care to homeopathic remedies to pharmacological interventions) through which they might intervene in such symptoms: rhetorics surrounding menopause, thus, appear relatively repetitive over time. To be fair, if Gunter's (2021) text is *The Silent Passage* of a new generation of menopausal women, it does move beyond Sheehy's (1992) in its openly anti-misogynist, overtly feminist messaging; its more frequent nods to marginalized person's experiences; and its stance that women are capable adults who are too often infantilized victims of patriarchy when it comes to their bodies, but they can arm themselves with information and advocate for themselves so that menopause can be a new beginning.

Even with these updates and progressions, though, texts about menopause often include a trope-like narrative arc on women experiencing symptoms, seeking support or care, and finding relief; this genre is plentiful. Such is the pattern of Heather Corinna's (2021) and Katie Muir's (2022) recent books. In the popular opinion or *doxa* that menopause is an unsolved riddle between disease and natural process, the message that women can't find good information or support persists over time *even as texts offering a wealth of knowledge and advice proliferate and have been around and plentiful for decades*. This message that women need more information and support to endure menopause continues to be put forward as a novel contribution, and the consequences of this erroneous claim are less space and attention given to misogyny and ageism as they characterize women's experiences with menopause. This is even true, we argue, of more progressive TikTok content on menopause that narrowly focuses on symptoms and treatments rather than taking up stigma explicitly.

To delve further into this topic, we use a corpus of recent texts that appear to be part of what some authors call a "menopause renaissance" to show how the *doxa* or popular opinion surrounding menopause leads to the perpetual claim that interest in menopause is somehow new and that more attention and less silence will lead to less suffering. The tension inherent in the trope of "menopause as/is a new concern" constitutes the undertow of diverse menopause texts, and while listing symptoms and potential remedies is a good thing, giving basic information on perimenopause and menopause is helpful, and women's stories have value in helping others to feel less alone and to even empower women to advocate for themselves, other potential intended agendas are lost or even hindered. Efforts at destigmatizing, of opening up space for more dialogue, and of promoting women's wellbeing above patriarchal concerns for preserving a highly heteronormative variety of youthful sex appeal are not achieved. Interrogating the fear of aging women and the idea that menopause is a harbinger of decline and death is not accomplished. What's worse, ironically, is that the trope of menopause as a new concern that is neither a medical disease nor a natural process, but something in-between that is a matter of symptoms and remedies, renders stigma potentially worsened by failing to ever adequately challenge the pervasive idea that menopause is really, at base, an unpleasant passage from youthful vitality to crone-like decrepitude.

Menopause is not an information and support wasteland, but it is still very much a dreaded concept associated with being put out to pasture. We, therefore, argue that rhetorics surrounding menopause are stuck in a loop that functions like this: an influential writer laments that women don't know enough about menopause and that something must be done to destigmatize the topic, a plethora of texts offering up that presumed missing information emerges, the tide of texts slows, and the process starts over—without, importantly, ever managing to dislodge or even nudge the misogyny and stigma that creates the silences in the first place—the dominant and utterly absurd view that there is shame and personal failure in aging and eventually even dying, particularly for women. This disposition is embedded so deeply in *doxa* that it is largely invisible. Efforts to increase awareness about menopause loop around the new information trope without ever touching this sexism.

This chapter also addresses the dearth of interest in the field of RHM on this topic. The omission of older women's experiences and the robust coverage of all things "reproductive" in the field had also come up in a conversation with rhetoric scholar Angela Crow, whose work has examined aging and literacies (2006). As a way of learning more about the readily available texts women might encounter in this significant phase of life, we collected key, representative texts in an intentional corpus at a moment in time. Below, we describe our approach to building out and analyzing our corpus of texts related to this topic such that our larger argument is clearer.

Methods and methodologies

Our method of data collection, as we mention above, made use of Kristi Cole and Anna Carmon's (2019) adaptation of Han Park's (2003) "observation on a hyperlinked network" (p. 293) to build a corpus of text for analysis. Following this method, we began with a *New York Times* article we'd all come across and clicked the hyperlinks and suggested related articles until we'd exhausted all links and/or until material began to repeat. Likewise, we used a Google news story search to find similar texts in publications outside of the US and outside of mainstream women's experiences (using the search terms "about menopause" and clicking through several screens) and added texts and linked texts until themes and content began to repeat while paying attention to place of publication such that we included a diverse range of texts in terms of, for example, political leanings of a particular publication. Since our interest was in recent discursive constructions of menopause, we used a time frame limiter of two years as an exclusion criterion. Recognizing that, with a few fringe exceptions, nonbinary women, trans-women, and BIPOC women are not focal points of most of the popular texts about menopause—even if they are given passing mention—we also used search terms to make sure we were catching any recent publications that *did* explicitly and exclusively focus on these populations. After we finished gathering texts, we eliminated redundancies (texts from similar or the same publications with the same kind of content).

This approach led us to gather a corpus of 16 English language texts that we feel confident are *representative of* what a variety of women might find if they are looking for information on menopause in popular media in 2021.

Table 4.1 shows the author, title, source, and publication month and year for each text included in the corpus.

We openly acknowledge the limitations of our corpus and want to argue, again, that it is representative of the *themes and concepts explored* in a particular time frame in popular publications on menopause rather than an exhaustive account of all that is out there at this moment. That said, since it includes a range of issues and topics in publications that span the political spectrum, and since topics include marginalized groups, we are also confident that this corpus captures the kinds of texts diverse women might find in popular publications. These limitations lead us to argue that this is a starting point and that it could provide a useful methodological framework for further study of this crucial topic.

After we established the corpus, we prepared the texts for analysis by uploading them to Nvivo software such that we could run word frequency queries, the results of which can be found in Table 4.2. Next, we used the results of these queries to guide an initial round of coding with the aim of ascertaining the popular opinions that undergird these contemporary writings on menopause. For this coding, we performed concept coding (Saldaña, 2021, p. 152) on the corpus of texts such that we could capture any themes that did not meaningfully emerge in word frequency queries. Results in the form of a final coding scheme can be found in Table 4.3. To capture other codes with less density but with significance, we also include Table 4.4, which shows codes with fewer than nine references that we still found important.

Methodologically, we approached analysis in a way that resembles critical discourse analysis (CDA) via a theoretical orientation to *doxa* as a guiding principle, meaning we thought about how the texts in our corpus worked to establish and perpetuate what is "considered true, or at least probable, by a majority of people endowed with reason, or by a specific social group" (Amossy, 2002, p. 369) with a consideration of these texts as constituting "a form of social practice" wherein "all social practices … are the means by which existing social relations are reproduced or contested and different interests are served" (Janks, 1997, p. 329).

Thus, we sought to uncover the "discursive undercurrents" (Gibbons, 2014, p. 445) that do significant epistemological work below the surface of discourses surrounding menopause, to categorize the major assumptions within these discourses, and to describe the potential material consequences of this *doxa* as it dictates inventional resources for the sources of information and forms of support that are available to peri- and post-menopausal women. Again, the most significant results of coding can be found in Table 4.3, and items coded with less density (which we operationalized as fewer than ten instances of that theme in the corpus) appear in Table 4.4. We included codes with nine or fewer references to show that these themes did emerge in the data, but we wanted to distinguish between these items and those that appeared with more density.

Table 4.1 Corpus of texts used in analysis

Author	Title	Source	Publication month/year
Jen Gunter	Women Can Have a Better Menopause. Here's How.	*New York Times*	May 2021
Jaclyn Friedman	'Who Knows When My Period Will Arrive Next?': A Frank Conversation about Menopause	*The Guardian*	June 2021
Sumathi Reddy	The Surprising Good News on How Menopause Changes Your Brain	*The Wall Street Journal Magazine*	June 2021
Lane Florsheim	Is the Menopause Product Boom Finally Here?	*The Wall Street Journal Magazine*	August 2020
Ashley Lauretta	What Can You Expect From Menopause? Here Are the Signs, Symptoms and Complications of Estrogen Loss	*Parade*	June 2021
Marlene Cimons	As Menopause Approaches, Some Women Suffer 'Brain Fog' and Memory Loss. What's Causing These Problems?	*The Washington Post*	May 2021
Jackie Gillard	Why Everyone Needs To Know More about Menopause — Especially Now	*The Washington Post*	June 2020
Sarah Vander Schaaff	Black Women's Health Problems during Menopause Haven't Been a Focus of Medicine. Experts and Activists Want to Change That.	*The Washington Post*	March 2021
Lisa Selin Davis	Why Modern Medicine Keeps Overlooking Menopause	*The New York Times*	April 2021
Gemma Fullam	I Am Woman: Hear Me Roar the Truth About The Menopause	*Independent Ireland*	April 2021
Sylvia Thompson	'The Menopause Is Where Mental Health Was 10 Years Ago'	*The Irish Times*	May 2021
Paula Akpan	Why Research and Conversation about Menopause Is Letting Down Black and Asian People	*Good Housekeeping*	February 2021
Megan Sutton	We Need to Talk about The LGBTQ+ Menopause Experience	*Good Housekeeping*	February 2021

(Continued)

Table 4.1 (Continued)

Author	Title	Source	Publication month/year
Katie Muir	Mission Menopause: 'My Hormones Went off a Cliff – And I'm not Going to Be Ashamed'	*The Guardian*	May 2021
Harriet Gibsone	Young, Hot and Bothered: Going Through Menopause in My 30s	*The Guardian*	June 2021
Alison Underhill	Bath Cancer Patient's Early Menopause 'Stark and Raw'	*BBC News*	July 2021

As a way to analyze the words that came up frequently in the corpus with a critical conception of *doxa* in mind, we categorized them and found that most fit into one of four categories:

- definitional/informational
- symptoms
- interventions
- support

After performing this parsing, we found that the word "society" remained and determined, from revisiting specific places in the corpus where this word came up, that this word was used in relation to stigmas and taboos surrounding menopause. While Table 4.2 shows word frequencies with information on which variations of each word were used and how many times the word was found in the corpus, Table 4.5 shows the word frequency table parsed using these four main categories and with "society" representative of the theme of stigmas and taboos in the corpus.

Word frequencies analysis

As Table 4.5 shows, a significant part of the rhetorical project of the texts in our corpus is to provide **definitional and informational content** on menopause, which coincides with the assumption that readers do not know very much about this topic and need key terms, ideas, and concepts delineated. As such, articles discussed what menopause *is*—the cessation of menstrual periods, and give definitions for related terms, such as perimenopause—the period of transition leading up to menopause. They also discuss how hormones factor into the menopause transition, what risks (health risks, risk of cancer) go along with this stage of life; how menopause relates to bodily

Table 4.2 Word frequency table

Word	Count	Includes these variations
menopause	657	menopausal, menopause, menopause'
symptoms	134	symptom, symptoms
health	122	health, health'
hormones	102	hormonal, hormonally, hormone, hormones, hormones'
experiences	78	experience, experiences, experiment
need	78	need, needed, needing, needs
changes	77	change, changed, changes, changing
periods	72	periods, period, periods
hot	71	hot
aging	54	ageing, age, aged, ageing, ages, aging
doctor	52	doctor, doctors, doctors'
perimenopause	51	perimenopausal, perimenopause
helps	50	help, helped, helpful, helping, helps
medical	48	medical, medically, medication, medications, medics
working	47	work, worked, working, works
brain	46	brain, brains
old	45	old
talk	44	talk, talked, talking, talks, talk'
body	41	bodies, body
hrt	41	hrt
treatment	39	treatment, treatments
signs	38	sign, signed, signs
research	38	research, researchers, researching
cancer	38	cancer, cancers
issues	37	issue, issues
clinics	37	clinic, clinical, clinically, clinics
caring	37	care, cared, careful, cares, caring
wellness	37	well, wellness
product	36	product, production, productive, productivity, products
family	34	families, family
information	34	information, informative
early	33	early
healthcare	33	healthcare
want	32	want, wanted, wanting, wants
medicine	32	medicine, medicines
support	31	support, supporting, supportive, supports
patient	30	patient, patients
risk	30	risk, risks, risks
study	30	studies, study
conversation	29	conversation, conversations, conversions
society	29	society
depression	28	depressants, depressed, depression
flashes	28	flash, flashes
access	27	access, accessed, accessibility, accessible, accessing
advertising	27	advertise, advertisement, advertising
transition	26	transition, transitions
story	26	stories, story
understand	25	understand, understanding, understands

Table 4.3 Final coding scheme

Code/theme	Number of items coded
Cognitive and mental health issues	21
Coping strategies	15
HRTs	11
Need for support	10
Silence about menopause	13
Stigma	11
Symptoms	18

Table 4.4 Other codes with nine or fewer references

- Care provider issues/misdiagnosis
- Changed/changing self-perception
- Comorbidities
- Equating menopause to puberty
- Health disparities
- Heteronormativity
- Ignorance about menopause
- Low levels of help-seeking
- Menopause renaissance
- Need for more research
- New phase of life
- New research and treatment
- Social determinants of health (SDOH)

aging/getting older; and the research/studies that have been done related to menopause, including exceptional cases (i.e., early menopause).

Another sizable portion of texts in our corpus was devoted to describing the signs and **symptoms** of menopause, such as cognitive/brain changes; mental health issues such as depression; bodily changes and experiences; hot flashes/flushes; and changing physical and mental health needs. The supposition, of course, is that readers will not be familiar with the signs and symptoms of menopause and will benefit from hearing a variety of them, making them better able to identify or recognize them in their own experiences, past and present, or anticipate them in the future.

Additionally, **interventions** meant to alleviate these signs and symptoms of menopause for women seeking help were covered vigorously in this corpus with references to healthcare and medical interventions, to access to care, and to doctors, patients, and clinics. Articles also mentioned products related to menopause and how they are advertised as well as whether or not various interventions work. In addition to interventions, these texts also focused on forms of support that women want beyond interventions, using words like talk, caring, wellness, family, support, conversation, and understanding.

Table 4.5 Word frequencies table by category

Category	Words
Definitional/informational	• menopause • perimenopause • early • story • health • hormones • information • risk • study • transition • aging • old • research • cancer • periods
Symptoms	• symptoms • changes • needs • hot • flashes • experiences • signs • brain • body • depression • issues
Interventions	• doctor • helps • medical • working • clinics • products • healthcare • patient • medicine • advertising • access
Support	• talk • caring • wellness • want • family • support • conversation • understand
Stigmas/taboos	• society

Naturally, the parts of these texts that talked about forms of **support** were at least tacitly activist in nature, indicating that women should get this support via menopause becoming more frequently talked about and considered. As we mention above, the word "society," while it didn't fit our basic four category breakdown of frequent words, appeared with significant density in this corpus, leading us to consider that another part of the rhetorical project of the texts included in this recent "menopause renaissance" is to destigmatize menopause and to remove taboos such that it enters more naturally into everyday conversations and women do not feel alone, confused, and misunderstood when they begin to experience signs and symptoms of the menopause transition. However, while efforts at destigmatization appear in the corpus, this focus is not new; such content has been present in menopausal discourses for decades as is evidenced in the introduction to this chapter. Yet menopause remains heavily stigmatized.

Taken together, what we notice examining word frequencies is that the popular opinion or *doxa* of menopause that emerges in this corpus is that it is a confusing transitional embodied experience that women do not understand when it starts to happen to them; thus, it is best addressed through being on the lookout for signs and symptoms and then advocating for the best care and support available. This epistemological undertow leads to the perpetual claim that interest in menopause is new and elides considerations of more activist agendas that could be taken up on this topic, such as how to make a real impact on the stigmas and taboos that follow it via calling out the misogynistic and ageist agendas that render it unintelligible and irrelevant in the first place. This epistemological undertow also leads to the idea that perimenopause and menopause are personal and individual when they are, instead, collected, communal, and always already happening.

Mapping word frequencies analysis to coding scheme

To advance our exploration of *doxa* and to further substantiate our argument that the *doxa* undergirding this corpus positions menopause as a fraught liminal state of being best addressed via individual preparation for symptoms and determinations of interventions, leading to the perpetual claim that interest in menopause is new and that stigmas and taboos surrounding it are best addressed via information, we explore how this word frequencies analysis maps to the data coding we also performed. In Table 4.6, we tagged each of our main codes with the category from our word frequencies analysis that each code fits with. That is, we found that our basic analytic framework for examining word frequencies mostly mapped to our concept coding scheme with some codes fitting "Symptoms" (Cognitive and mental health issues; Symptoms), some fitting "Interventions" (Coping strategies; HRTs); some fitting "Support" (Need for support), and some fitting "Stigmas and taboos" (Silence about menopause; Stigma). While our coding scheme did not reveal

Table 4.6 Coding scheme with themes from word frequencies noted

Code/theme	Number of items coded
Cognitive and mental health issues (symptoms)	21
Coping strategies (interventions)	15
HRTs (interventions)	11
Need for support (support)	10
Silence about menopause (stigmas and taboos)	13
Stigma (stigmas and taboos)	11
Symptoms (symptoms)	18

the informational/definitional content of the corpus as effectively as the word frequencies did, it does substantiate our claim that this is a discourse that is stuck in a loop. That is, it makes it clear that the themes that emerge in popular texts about menopause are highly repetitive.

Accounting for coding categories with less density

There were several concept coding categories that did emerge in our corpus, yet with less significant density than the items that appeared in our main coding scheme. These items, though, still are interesting trends to consider in the rhetorical landscape of menopause during this "menopause renaissance." Like the word frequencies analysis, some of these items map to the category of "Informational/definitional," such as claims that we are in a "menopause renaissance;" equating menopause to puberty; ignorance about menopause; new research and treatment; and comorbidities.

That said, the fact that some of the more critical commentary represented in these codes make up less of a significant presence in the corpus also helps us to account for how and why the more activist, anti-misogyny arguments get lost in the midst of the more dominant content to do with information, symptoms, treatments, and supports. These include health disparities; issues with care providers, including the misdiagnosis of menopause-related symptoms; heteronormativity; the need for more research; and social determinants of health (SDOHs). Likewise, some of these less dense codes speak to women's dispositions toward menopause, such as a changed or changing self-perception; the sense that one is entering a new phase of life; and how these things might lead to low levels of help-seeking. The fact that these more critical and self-perceptual items appeared in the data, but with less significant density than items related to symptoms, interventions, and support shows us two things: First, we can ascertain that concerns for how intersectional marks of difference impact the menopause transition are out there. However, we also find that concerns for how race, socioeconomic status, and gender impact menopause are easily overshadowed by the persuasive message that the real issue women face when encountering this health flashpoint is lack of information. In menopause discourses, marginalized individuals get inadequate attention, and the pervasive assumption of socioeconomic privilege, of heterosexuality, and of cisgendered personhood is quite obvious.

Analysis

Our analysis leads us to argue that the *doxa* that undergirds recent texts on menopause is that it is a liminal state of being shrouded in mystery that is best addressed via individual determinations of interventions, leading to the perpetual claim that interest in menopause is new even as texts about menopause that say remarkably similar things can be traced back decades. This newness argument, we contend, has the unintended consequence of stagnating the public discourse surrounding menopause, leaving stigma intact, and continuing to pay homage to ciscentric, heteronormative, patriarchal ideas about women and aging—that women going through menopause are rightly bothered by the loss of traditional femininity, that the height of womanhood is synonymous with ovaries, periods, pregnancies, and breasts, etc., and that individual women must take responsibility for mitigating the negative consequences of misogyny in everyday life via individual acts of self-care and self-advocacy related to menopause.

As we note above, collectively, these texts share didactic purposes—to teach women to spot the symptoms of perimenopause, menopause, and postmenopause; to instruct women on when to proactively alter lifestyle, habits, routines, etc. to prepare for this transition; and to empower women to seek care and insist on the best interventions possible given the most recent and rigorous science. Yet these purposes don't further the more pressing activist women's health agenda—to make all aging women (Black and Brown women, transwomen, nonbinary persons with uteruses, socioeconomically disadvantaged women, disabled women) and their health matter more in the public sphere and to mitigate ageism and misogyny that lead to erasure and indifference. This activist project also needs to be accounted for in RHM literature itself where coverage of aging women's health is far lower in contrast to a wealth of scholarship on the rhetoric of reproduction.

Rhetorics of menopause as agnotology

In some ways, our discussion of rhetorics of menopause resembles how Judy Segal (2007) used agnotology, or "the study of the cultural production of ignorance" (p. 4) to explore how the genre of the breast cancer narrative contributes to misinformation about breast cancer. "This is my agnotology thesis," Segal wrote: "Personal breast cancer stories are one means of producing and maintaining ignorance about breast cancer. They do this, in part, generically" (2007, p. 4).

Just as Segal saw promise in agnotology as a conceptual frame through which to explore how cultural ignorance about breast cancer is created via the standard cancer story—that it is a predictable, linear journey with a happy ending—we see promise in agnotology as a conceptual frame to account for how menopause texts that narrowly focus on definitions, signs, symptoms, interventions, and supports might contribute to cultural ignorance surrounding menopause rather than doing the work that advocates and activists want these discourses to be doing, which we claim is to dismantle the patriarchal invisibility of diverse older women, their bodies, their concerns, and their futures. Whereas Segal saw genre as operative in the creation of cultural ignorance related to breast cancer, we see this happening with menopause on the level of topics of coverage and at the level of *doxa* as a powerful perpetuating force that operates imperfectively below the surface of discourse.

Unpacking menopause doxa: neurotic loops

As our analysis shows, too, anyone looking for information on menopause that will give basic definitional information, describe common symptoms, and overview potential interventions will not have to look far to find what they want. That said, the *doxa* that serves as the undercurrent for this discourse is that if women were better informed, they'd seek care for treatable symptoms and emerge from this temporary, albeit unpleasant, phase of life better off. This popular opinion ignores the fact that for many, information—even very good, timely, cutting-edge, data-driven, feminist, helpful information—isn't enough to undercut the various ways that women, and especially women of color, are disenfranchised in medical encounters and beyond and that aging women are a feared and hated group.

What's more, efforts to bring awareness to menopause as a phenomenon, to offer symptom alleviation/relief, and to regularize talking about it have not impacted stigma surrounding it in any meaningful way. This has led to a perpetual loop of texts claiming that concerns about menopause are new when they are not new at all and are, in fact, quite prolific and influential in their *doxastic* way. Discourses around menopause have, thus, created what we would even call their own neurotic loops that stagnate health discourses even as they do offer, at times, individual women readers the sense that they are not alone, some indication of what they could do for their symptoms, and some hope that they will regain their lives. "Neurotic loops," explained Gregg Henriques (2019) are critical reactions to negative feelings that lead to more negative feelings, followed by more critical reactions, and so on. In the same way, the health flashpoint of menopause leads to negative feelings that feed critical reactions that never, via available discourses, break out of more negative affect since that effect has its origins in misogyny and not, as the discourse would suggest, in lack of information. Crucially, as well, even these sources of information and forms of support are paltry for marginalized and multiply marginalized women who'll find themselves at the fringe of the robust, repeating discourses surrounding menopause, which are mainly aimed at a heteronormative, white, and socioeconomically advantaged subset of the population—those with the ability to advocate for themselves, to carefully choose care providers, to have the luxury of time and space to test out remedies, etc. That is to say that this narrative of "if patients were better informed, things could improve" always already presupposes a number of racial, socioeconomic class, and gender privileges, and information—even very good information—can only do so much for certain people.

Menopause, it should be emphasized, is still shrouded in silence, still not a part of everyday conversation. More importantly, as Susan Sontag's (1972) coinage "the double standard of aging" continues to demonstrate in newer iterations, older women are still despised, feared, ignored, and invisible (Åberg et al., 2020), and the impulse to ignore, fear, and despise aging women will be, of course, much more pronounced for women with other compounding forms of marginalization. These realities are the crucial ones that need more attention in the discourses surrounding menopause.

Resisting the undercurrent: some promising places for alternative forms of support and sources of information

As Laurie McMillan (2019) argued, there are times when advocacy work related to women's health can appear, on the surface, to be in the service of long-range feminist agendas, yet ironically undercut such efforts; her work showed how short-term activism can sometimes hurt the long game. We feel the same way about some forms of support we see emerging in the midst of this "menopause renaissance," such as the existence of "menopause midwives." Not everything, we'd argue, in women's health should be a metaphor for birth and birthing, and the idea of midwifery for menopause does just that. As Bryna commented on the promises or perils of the idea of a menopause midwife, "She can hang out with me in the middle of the night when I'm wide awake sweating to death." In the same way, equating menopause with puberty is not helpful because puberty is often explained to young people explicitly and is seen as a new and hopeful phase of life for all people (not just one gender) that is highly anticipated (with its good and bad aspects of course).

Solving the riddle, then, of how to approach menopause rhetorics with an aim of dismantling stigma and misogyny are beyond the scope of this chapter, yet we do want to conclude our analysis with some sources of information to check out if you want to see some more overtly activist content than what you'll find in the mainstream.

• Omisade Burney-Scott's multimedia activist project "The Black Girl's Guide to Surviving Menopause"

- Karen Arthur's "Menopause Whilst Black" podcast
- Davina McCall's documentary "Sex, Myths, and the Menopause"
- Sallyanne Brady's "The Irish Menopause" project
- Heather Dillaway and Laura Wershler's (2021) edited collection *Musings on Perimenopause and Menopause: Identity, Experience, Transition*

We'd further recommend using Gunter's (2021) book as an accessible reference text (the index is your friend) when you have a specific question related to a particular symptom or treatment—especially if you need to know what recent research says about the risks to benefit ratio of a particular drug.

Breaking out of neurotic loops: rhetorical enactments of menopause as future research direction

Tending to the undercurrent of misogyny as it relates to the more pressing issues menopause raises is possible with a consideration of rhetorical enactments. Molly Kessler (2020) defined rhetorical enactments as "a theoretical frame that attunes to how entities such as mind, body, self, and non-self are enacted in space and time through practice, and how such enactments are made meaningful;" rhetorical enactments "shift the analytic focus away from perspectives about" a phenomenon "toward practices and experiences that rhetorically enact multiple" instantiations of that phenomenon (p. 298). Showing the limitations of focusing on patients' attitudes and perspectives and arguing that such focal points leave space to say that patients' experiences can improve if they change their thinking, Kessler puts forward rhetorical enactments as a way to attune to how ostomies are staged in a "constellation of practices" and, thus, allows for the possibility that the practices themselves can be shifted (2020, p. 317). As we contemplate what resources exist for more effective menopause activism, Kessler's work leads us to ask: How is menopause staged in ways that move outside the range of definitions, symptoms, interventions, and support that might point beyond perspectives and attitudes of the individual? Future work could take up rhetorical enactments as they relate to menopause to further explore this health flashpoint—particularly as enactments offer an alternative to narrative tropes. In the intervening time, we hope all women in the midst of the health flashpoints of menopause critically evaluate the claim that it is an unpleasant experience simply due to lack of information.

References

Åberg, E., Kukkonen, I., & Sarpila, O. (2020). From double to triple standards of ageing: Perceptions of physical appearance at the intersections of age, gender and class. *Journal of Aging Studies*, *55*, 1–12. https://doi.org/10.1016/j.jaging.2020.100876

Akpan, P. (2021, February 16). Why research and conversation about menopause is letting down Black and Asian people. *Good Housekeeping.* https://www.goodhousekeeping.com/uk/health/a35000306/menopause-research-healthcare-letting-down-black-and-asian-people/

Amossy, R. (2002). Introduction to the study of doxa. *Poetics Today, 23*(3), 369–394. https://doi.org/10.1215/03335372-23-3-369

Arthur, K. (Host). (2020–present). *Menopause whilst Black* [Audio podcast]. https://www.thekarenarthur.com/menopausewhilstblack

Brady, S. (n.d.). *The Irish Menopause.* http://www.theirishmenopause.com

Burney-Scott, O. (n.d.). *Black girl's guide to surviving menopause.* https://blackgirlsguidetosurvivingmenopause.com/#about

Chrisler, J. C. (2011). Leaks, lumps, and lines: Stigma and women's bodies. *Psychology of Women Quarterly, 35*(2), 202–214. https://doi.org/10.1177/0361684310397698

Cimons, M. (2021, May 16). As menopause approaches, some women suffer 'brain fog' and memory loss. What's causing these problems? *Washington Post.* https://www.washingtonpost.com/health/brain-fog-menopause-memory-loss/2021/05/14/0600c088-aea6-11eb-ab4c-986555a1c511_story.html

Cole, K. L., & Carmon, A. F. (2019). Changing the face of the opioid epidemic: A generic rhetorical analysis of addiction obituaries. *Rhetoric of Health & Medicine, 2*(3), 291–320. https://doi.org/10.5744/rhm.2019.1014

Corinna, H. (2021). *What fresh hell is this? Perimenopause, menopause, other indignities, and you.* Hachette Books.

Crow, A. (2006). *Aging literacies: Training and development challenges for faculty.* Hampton Press.

Dillaway, H., & Wershler, L. (Eds.). (2021). *Musings on perimenopause and menopause: Identity, experience, transition.* Demeter.

Dominus, S. (2023, February 1). Women have been misled about menopause. *New York Times.* https://www.nytimes.com/2023/02/01/magazine/menopause-hot-flashes-hormone-therapy.html

Florsheim, L. (2020, August 25). Is the menopause product boom finally here? *Wall Street Journal Magazine.* https://www.wsj.com/articles/is-the-menopause-product-boom-finally-here-11598367930

Friedman, J. (2021, June 21). 'Who knows when my period will arrive next?': A frank conversation about menopause. *The Guardian.* https://www.theguardian.com/lifeandstyle/2021/jun/21/menopause-conversation-people-want-to-capitalize-on-us-ageing-

Fullam, G. (2021, May 16). I am woman: Hear me roar the truth about the menopause. *Independent Ireland.* https://www.independent.ie/opinion/comment/i-am-woman-hear-me-roar-the-truth-about-the-menopause/40430326.html

Gibbons, M. G. (2014). Beliefs about the mind as doxastic inventional resource: Freud, neuroscience, and the case of Dr. Spock's "Baby and Child Care." *Rhetoric Society Quarterly, 44*(5), 427–448. https://doi.org/10.1080/02773945.2014.957411

Gibsone, H. (2021, June 27). Young, hot and bothered: Going through menopause in my 30s. *The Guardian.* https://www.theguardian.com/news/audio/2021/jun/28/young-hot-and-bothered-going-through-menopause-in-my-30s

Gillard, J. (2020, June 29). Why everyone needs to know more about menopause—Especially now. *Washington Post.* https://www.washingtonpost.com/lifestyle/

wellness/why-everyone-needs-to-know-more-about-menopause--especially-now
/2020/06/29/d0ec9f76-b7e2-11ea-aca5-ebb63d27e1ff_story.html

Gunter, J. (2021). *The menopause manifesto: Own your health with facts and feminism.* Citadel.

Gunter, J. (2021, May 25). Women can have a better menopause. *Here's How. New York Times.* https://www.nytimes.com/2021/05/25/opinion/feminist-menopause.html

Gupta, A. H. (2023, January 13). What is menopause like for women of color? *New York Times.* https://www.nytimes.com/2023/01/13/us/menopause-experiences.html

Henriques, G. (2019, June 5). What to do if you are depressed: Identify neurotic loops. *Psychology Today.* https://www.psychologytoday.com/us/blog/theory-knowledge /201906/what-do-if-you-are-depressed-identify-neurotic-loops

Houck, J. A. (2003). "What do these women want?" Feminist responses to Feminine Forever, 1963–1980. *Bulletin of the History of Medicine, 77*(1), 103–132. https:// doi.org/10.1353/bhm.2003.0023

Janks, H. (1997). Critical discourse analysis as a research tool. *Discourse: Studies in the Cultural Politics of Education, 18*(3), 329–342. https://doi.org/10.1080 /0159630970180302

Kessler, M. M. (2020). The ostomy multiple: Toward a theory of rhetorical enactments. *Rhetoric of Health & Medicine, 3*(3), 293–319. https://doi.org/10.5744/rhm.2020 .1016

Larocca, A. (2022, December 21). Welcome to the menopause gold rush. *New York Times.* https://www.nytimes.com/2022/12/20/style/menopause-womens-health-goop .html

Lauretta, A. (2021, June 30). *What can you expect from menopause? Here are the signs, symptoms and complications of estrogen loss.* Parade. https://parade.com/1229756/ ashleylauretta/what-is-menopause/

Matlock, B. (2021). Moving the story forward utilizing deminer narratives to increase women's empowerment in mine action and beyond. *The Journal of Conventional Weapons Destruction, 25*(1). https://commons.lib.jmu.edu/cisr-journal/vol25/iss1 /14

McMillan, L. (2019). Costly expedience: Reproductive rights and responses to slut shaming. In J. White-Farnham, B. Siegel Finer, & C. Molloy (Eds.), *Women's health advocacy: Rhetorical ingenuity for the 21st century* (pp. 191–203). Routledge.

Muir, K. (2021, May 9). Mission menopause: 'My hormones went off a cliff – and I'm not going to be ashamed.' *The Guardian.* https://www.theguardian.com/society /2021/may/09/mission-menopause-my-hormones-went-off-a-cliff-and-im-not -going-to-be-ashamed

Muir, K. (2022). *Everything you need to know about the menopause.* Gallery UK.

Nosek, M., Kennedy, H. P., Beyene, Y., Taylor, D., Gilliss, C., & Lee, K. (2010). The effects of perceived stress and attitudes toward menopause and aging on symptoms of menopause. *Journal of Midwifery and Women's Health, 55*(4), 328–334. https:// doi.org/10.1016/j.jmwh.2009.09.005

Park, H. (2003). Hyperlink network analysis: A new method for the study of social structure on the web. *Connections, 25*, 49–61.

Reddy, S. (2021, June 14). The surprising good news on how menopause changes your brain. *The Wall Street Journal Magazine.* https://www.wsj.com/articles/the -surprising-good-news-on-how-menopause-changes-your-brain-11623698003#

Saldaña, J. (2021). *The coding manual for qualitative researchers* (4th ed.). SAGE Publications.

Sands, L. (Director). (2021). *Davina McCall: Sex, myths and the menopause* [Documentary]. Channel 4 Television. United Kingdom.

Segal, J. Z. (2008). Breast cancer narratives as public rhetoric: Genre itself and the maintenance of ignorance. *Linguistics and the Human Sciences, 3*(1), 3–23. https://doi.org/10.1558/lhs.v3i1.3

Selin Davis, L. (2021, April 6). Why modern medicine keeps overlooking menopause. *New York Times.* https://www.nytimes.com/2021/04/06/us/menopause-perimenopause-symptoms.html

Sheehy, G. (1992). *The silent passage.* Random House.

Siegel Finer, B. (2019). Afterword: "The rhetorician [of health and medicine] as agent of social change": Activism for the whole woman's body. In J. White-Farnham, B. Siegel Finer, & C. Molloy (Eds.), *Women's health advocacy: Rhetorical ingenuity for the 21st century* (pp. 204–212). Routledge.

Sontag, S. (1972). The double standard of aging. *Saturday Review of Literature, 39*(1), 29–38.

Sutton, M. (2021, February 16). We need to talk about the LGBTQ+ menopause experience. *Good Housekeeping.* https://www.goodhousekeeping.com/uk/health/a35227597/lgbtq-menopause-experience/

Syme, M. L., & Cohn, T. J. (2016). Examining aging sexual stigma attitudes among adults by gender, age, and generational status. *Aging and Mental Health, 20*(1), 36–45. https://doi.org/10.1080/13607863.2015.1012044

Thompson, S. (2021, May 15). The menopause is where mental health was 10 years ago. *The Irish Times.* https://www.irishtimes.com/life-and-style/health-family/the-menopause-is-where-mental-health-was-10-years-ago-1.4564003#:~:text=Loretta%20Dignam%2C%20who%20set%20up,health%20was%2010%20years%20ago"

Underhill, A. (2021, July 2). Bath cancer patient's early menopause "stark and raw." *BBC News.* https://www.bbc.com/news/uk-england-somerset-57664465

Vander Schaaff, S. (2021, March 6). Black women's health problems during menopause haven't been a focus of medicine. Experts and activists want to change that. *Washington Post.* https://www.washingtonpost.com/health/black-women-menopause-hot-flashes/2021/03/05/97a02c44-7b8a-11eb-a976-c028a4215c78_story.html

Wilson, R. (1966). *Feminine forever: A new life, the quest and the key.* M Evans & Co.

5   Making sense of sobriety as a woman

Expanding options for patient epistemologies

In the last chapter, we demonstrated that forms of support are heavily dependent on material realities and socioeconomic status and that rhetorical work can be limited by what is present in popular opinion, uncritically accepted traditions, dominant narratives, and *doxa*. Taking a turn from the discourses of menopause, this chapter is about how sobriety animates the process of patient epistemologies with examples of promising changes to the field of discourse available to women at the health flashpoint of seeking sobriety.

Sobriety discourses have been long dominated by the lore and practices of Alcoholics Anonymous (AA), including the "Twelve Steps," which are instantiated in the amateur self-help realm, the professional sphere, and the popular imagination. AA has been well-critiqued for its male-centric, Christian origins and emphases, and attempts to revise and temper these elements of AA for a female audience do exist. That said, the alternatives do not always have the rhetorical heft they'd need to displace the hegemony of AA, and the *doxa* in support of AA is pervasive. This chapter analyzes a text that works to adapt AA to women's needs as well as a notable recent alternative text. We aim to show how and why this alternative text lends itself to improved cycles of patient epistemologies when women seek sobriety.

A casual perusal of popular sobriety discourses suggests that AA is the main and perhaps only option so that those who are marginalized in AA episteme should adapt the program to their needs. However, based on the work of feminist scholars, activists, and everyday women to understand and create varieties and types of discourses that reflect women's lived experiences, the available means for recovery and maintaining sobriety have expanded. And while the expansion has not (and probably cannot and will not) totally dislodged AA hegemony, the creation and existence of alternative discourses shows that change to *doxa* is possible. This chapter traces the expansion of women's sobriety discourses over time by comparing the conceptual frameworks of two popular women's sobriety texts: *A Woman's Way Through the Twelve Steps* (AWW) by Stephanie Covington (1994) and *Quit Like a Woman* (QLAW) (2021) by Holly Whitaker.

We contend that in presenting a new rhetorical framework for alcoholism, Whitaker has done something imaginative and quite difficult to do, as our

DOI: 10.4324/9781003398318-5

menopause discourse analysis shows. *QLAW* takes the onus off of the individual's addiction to alcohol and places blame and action for improvement on the large and profitable alcohol industry, or "Big Alcohol"—something akin to "Big Tobacco." Our analysis of her and Covington's texts shows that while some messages related to health proliferate and dominate the discourse unchecked, alternatives exist and can support multiple epistemologies. To support our analysis of these texts, Jamie also provides first-hand rhetorical encounters with conflicting and inadequate discourses upon being inducted into the rhetorical community of sobriety herself. By way of conclusion, we use our analysis of the narrative-centric discourses of recovery to suggest a continued expansion of rhetorical frameworks that might be added to the explicit options for discourses, epistemological tools, and forms of support for women in recovery.

Methodology for tracing expansions of sobriety discourses

In the early days of Jamie's sobriety, her treatment counselor guessed right away, based on demographics of gender, age, religious preference, and education, that she might be interested in *A Woman's Way Through the Twelve Steps*, a book that acknowledges the male-centric wording and concepts that do not sit easily with empowered women, including powerlessness (step 1) and turning one's life over (step 3). The counselor was correct, and Jamie *was* interested in that interpretation, but still found the discourses of AA, even recast for women, lacking. In important ways, her rhetorical work at this health flashpoint felt limited to the pervasive message that AA is the only way to obtain and maintain sobriety. In reading this text and searching for other relevant accounts of women's sobriety that might be helpful, Jamie couldn't help but notice the limits and affordances of what Emily Hogg (2019) called "stock narratives" about alcoholism in our culture, such as the "drunkard narrative" and the "cautionary tale" (Hogg, 2019, pp. 315–316). Importantly, neither of these described Jamie's nor many women's experiences with alcoholism, and Hogg asserts that resistance to stock narratives emerges because of "their inability to tell individual and distinctive stories" (2019, p. 311).

Jamie searched for something else on the internet with terms like "sobriety and moms," "Gen X sobriety" or "feminist sobriety." Eventually, she came across various blogs and social media groups, including "Hip Sobriety"—a blog that did not endorse a prescribed approach to sobriety and did not align with AA. Hip Sobriety was founded by *Quit Like a Woman* author Holly Whitaker (the site predates the book by a number of years), whose understanding of sobriety was appealing as it presented an alternative to the "rock bottom" narrative: "you don't need to hit rock bottom." As Anne Dowsett-Johnston (2014) and also Hogg (2019) point out, many women do not exhibit a public downfall when they are alcoholics, such as hitting rock bottom or getting a DUI. In fact, although Jamie was gratified to find "Hip Sobriety" and the general concept of "sobriety without AA," the path to AA alternatives was not clear. Without advanced information literacies, we wondered, how is this rhetoric work undertaken at this particular health flashpoint, and how can such alternatives be made more legible to the general public?

The two texts for women seeking sobriety at the focus of this chapter present interesting polarities and tensions produced by their arguments and assumptions. While *A Woman's Way* helps women to adapt AA to women's needs, *Quit Like a Woman* encourages women to, instead, conceptualize their experiences with alcohol within the larger context of the cultural pressure of Big Alcohol. We chose these texts to help us to theorize how alternatives to deeply entrenched *doxa* might operate and how they might be made to better proliferate. The former text takes the position that AA is the preferred or even only viable way to get sober but allows that it needs specific interpretation to better fit a woman's needs. The latter challenges the *doxa* not only of AA but of definitions of alcoholism itself.

Methodologically, our analysis in this chapter relies on the principles of Kathleen J. Ryan's (2010) feminist textual methodology, including such features as:

- sharing work within a frame of polarizing paired arguments, which makes space for "more entangled discussions," offering to the feminist conversation something which can further be complicated, rather than settled (p. 95). This feature of Ryan's methodology made our choice of texts clear— *A Woman's Way* and *Quit Like a Woman* do present us with a fitting polarizing pair such that we might further complicate sources of information and forms of support at women's health flashpoints.
- bringing voices to the scholarly conversation that might not otherwise be there. This act, to Ryan, "defines and broadens fields of inquiry, while at the same time identifying issues that demand attention" (Hawisher & Selfe, as cited in Ryan, 2019, p. 95). Popular self-help books related to women's sobriety, while somewhat unlikely as scholarly artifacts, deserve more scholarly attention, we argue.

Our process of analysis contributes to the continuing project of feminist research methodologies by drawing on lived experience as a valid and important source of knowledge and understanding.

We also focused our analysis on the role narrative plays in each text. A review of related literature attests to the fact that much scholarly attention to the topic of women's sobriety has analyzed women's narratives (Hogg, 2019; Lund, 2016; Prussing, 2007). Narrative is a well-known and established rhetorical and healing tool in the process of sobriety. It serves a constitutive function—("Hello, my name is ____, and I'm an alcoholic"); a therapeutic function that is well-documented in studies of writing and healing (see, for instance, Pennebaker, 1990; Anderson & MacCurdy, 2000, among others);

and a rhetorical function in its capacity to inspire and inform others who may be looking for their own starting point in sobriety. That is, by hearing a person share their journey of seeking sobriety, others who are struggling with substance use disorders might hear echoes of their own experiences in such narratives and see a way forward for themselves in the arcs presented. Recent feminist studies of available sobriety narratives reveal attempts at expansion from what Hogg (2019) called "stock narratives" of sobriety that are bound up in male-centric understandings of the identities and behaviors of an alcoholic. Hogg and others are seeking to offer narrative alternatives that reflect women's experiences as distinct from men; yet, they are still focused on narrative as the dominant rhetorical mode.

Both texts under analysis include narrative within them, though the multiple rhetorical tactics that exceed narration will also be unpacked. Whitaker, in fact, brings a novel argument to this discourse for what seems to be the first time. She empowers women to consider the forces and systems that created the conditions in which they have become dependent on alcohol in the first place, rather than rest on two main pillars of previous sobriety work: that the woman herself should be the focus of any critical thought about alcoholism and that all experiences regarding women and sobriety are by default a "narrative." We approached the analysis by reading through the books several times and charting notable trends that reveal *doxa* related to women and sobriety, the primacy of narrative, the hegemony of AA, and alternatives to these rigid positions.

Analysis of A Woman's Way Through the Twelve Steps, 1994 (AWW)

A Woman's Way Through the Twelve Steps by Stephanie Covington is a best-selling companion to the AA program published by Hazelden in 1994. Covington is a psychologist and expert on gender and trauma-informed approaches to addiction treatment. Our analysis of *AWW* considers the text as a net-positive contribution to sobriety discourse in its attempts to interpret the twelve steps explicitly for then-modern women of the 1990s. Rhetorically speaking, it includes some of the typical AA conventions of sharing personal experiences anonymously and using what Trysh Travis (2009) would call commonplaces, such as the Serenity Prayer and other pithy sayings. The book faces the logical difficulty of convincing women that a model made for, about, and by white, cisgender, heterosexual men (and never officially updated or revised for any other type of person) will work for them (but is still not for them, just will still also work for them). In essence, Covington's rhetorical project is to convince women that there is value in taking on a program that was never intended for them.

The book's purpose is clearly stated. Because AA was founded in 1939 and the twelve steps were written by men "at a time when women had few resources and little social, political, or power […], many of us [women] have struggled to stay with a recovery program that does not completely meet our needs or match our values" (1994, pp. 1–2). Covington thus offers "a more open exploration" and "a more flexible interpretation" of the twelve steps, organized with each chapter explaining a step, followed by chapters on the Self, Relationships, Sexuality, and Spirituality.

Showing her own adherence to the popular opinion that AA is the only way to achieve and maintain sobriety, Covington was not willing to overhaul the steps completely, noting that the original spirit of the program is important to maintain. She also argued that the steps may already be inherently feminine, in the sense that it is a mutual-aid program without hierarchy or authorities: "Rather than rewrite the Steps in a way that attempts to fit all women, we can instead work with the original Steps–paying close attention to the spirit and meaning–and reinterpreting the language to support our own recovery […] when we look inside ourselves and reframe the original wording in the way that works best for us, each of us, individually, can discover the meaning for ourselves" (Covington, 1994, p. 5). Our analysis of Covington's book revealed three key features we elaborate on below: the use of individual examples and stories; the use of growth metaphors; and the strategic embracing and erasing of contradictions.

Individual examples & stories

Generally speaking, the overall philosophy of the book suggests the value of fitting into the steps in an inviting and slow way, mulling over each step and considering Covington's many anecdotes and examples of women who have worked the steps to achieve sobriety:

> We all have more to offer than the party line and a by-the-book recitation of the Steps. We can share our story any way we like. As long as we're honest and sincere, we can't go wrong. It's as simple as saying, "This worked for me and it might work for you too."
>
> (Covington, 1994, p. 188)

Covington sees storytelling and story consumption as key features that make AA both successful and adaptable for women.

Covington's confidence in such story sharing and telling is evident in how the book is arranged; in fact, anecdotal examples that illustrate the ways women make connections across varying experiences are one of the main rhetorical features of the book. A typical example will follow Covington's interpretation of a step, offering illumination of her point and adding a complication, caveat, or nuance. In the best examples, Covington uses an expert therapist's nonjudgmental tone to apply the steps to various situations. For instance, consider an example of how the fifth step, admitting the exact nature of one's wrongs to another person, helped Mary Lynn when she shared her "wrongs" with a trusted person, Tanya:

> With Tanya, Mary Lynn was able to recount the experiences she felt most ashamed of: picking up men in bars, engaging in sex in front of her young children [...] in recovery, [Tanya] realized that she could live a life in which alcohol and drugs had no place and could refuse to have the kind of sex she didn't want. Even though the details of Tanya's story were different from Mary Lynn's, her experience told Mary Lynn "I've been there too."
>
> (Covington, 1994, p. 81)

Covington acknowledges 20 anonymous women for their participation in being interviewed for the book in her acknowledgment section, but the names used in the examples are, of course, pseudonyms. In addition, Covington herself uses her sobriety experience as examples often as well.

Growth metaphors

Another main rhetorical feature is metaphors about growth, and especially developmental comparisons of a newly sober person to a baby and to the lotus flower. To create a caring and nurturing approach to sobriety, perhaps rather than "tough love," Covington compares the process of getting sober to the development of babies, emphasizing that "just as an infant needs a safe, nurturing environment to grow and develop, so do we" (1994, p. 203) and that, during the process, when things get difficult, it is expected that a newly sober person might react like a baby who gets cranky right before hitting a big milestone, such as being frustrated one can't walk yet: "like this child, we're bound to get cranky and mad as hell when we know what we want to do but can't quite do it yet" (1994, p. 102). Through the infancy metaphor, Covington attempts to create a kinder version of the twelve steps such that women can see themselves represented in them.

The lotus is the most-used metaphor, and there is a painting of one on the book's cover accompanied by a brief explanation of its choice:

> I see the lotus as a symbol of women's recovery. Recovery is a transformational experience. When a woman recovers, she is able to say, "Who I am today is not who I was." The elegant and beautiful lotus flower that emerges from the mud is the beautiful woman within.
>
> (Covington, 1994, p. 6)

The contradiction of the flower and the mud is an important part of this metaphor, as the origins of the process of sobriety may be seen as "dirty" but necessary for the growth of the flower. Covington writes:

As recovering women, we are like the lotus flower, sending our roots down into the mud, our addiction, but always seeking the light. We, like the lotus, don't detach from the mud. Our spirituality is not found by separating ourselves from anything but by staying connected – to the mud, to the truth about our addiction, or to the reality of our life as the source that "grows us."

(1994, p. 230)

Readers will notice that the roots are a vital part of the lotus flower and, thus, the woman's past experiences with addiction are part of what make her the beautiful flower she is becoming.

Embracing/erasing contradictions

Beyond offering women a way to see their experiences with addiction as a necessary part of their life stories, the lotus' ability to communicate the concept of contradiction poetically and well is necessary for a reader to be able to orient herself to the many contradictions present in the book. Covington's purpose is to reinterpret and reify the steps, which often entails satisfying the reader that even though the text says X, it really means Y. While a rundown of each step is outside of the scope of this analysis, below we provide two examples of how Covington embraces contradictions and offers generous definitions of words in order to make palatable interpretations of the steps for women readers.

Two of the most feministly-critiqued concepts in the steps are admitting one was powerless (step 1) and surrendering oneself to God (step 3). For each, Covington lays a foundation for understanding why these steps were problematic to modern women in the 1990s. She writes of the first step:

The word powerlessness is a problem for many women. Many of us were taught to let something or someone else control our lives. It can be difficult to acknowledge we are powerless over our addictions because we already feel powerless in so many other areas of our lives.

(Covington, 1994, p. 12)

Yet, of course, the point of the book is to make this concept that might not make sense to its audience make some type of sense. Covington acknowledges that there is a paradox at play: "Yet only when we admit our powerlessness and lack of control over our addiction can we begin to find out where we truly have power in our lives" (1994, p. 12). In this manner, she is saying that women do have some power, but it is perhaps hidden or overshadowed by addiction at the moment. Once you do the first step and admit powerlessness, then you will have power: "Let powerlessness be your partner and guide you to a new experience of power. Awareness of unmanageability in your life is a sign that you are on the recovery path" (Covington, 1994, p. 25). Covington asks women to see powerlessness as actually, in the end, quite empowering—a move that does not so much address the powerlessness women feel in their everyday lives due to widespread sexism as it asks women to ignore systemic misogyny in favor of using the steps for their own ends. This tactic—embracing contradictions within the steps by allowing a word to mean its opposite—also occurs in the third step.

AA alternately refers to a Higher Power and God. Often, the higher power is emphasized as anything a person needs it to be, whether a deity of a certain religion, or something less-defined spiritually-speaking. However, the third step names God outright: "we made a decision to turn our will and our lives over to the care of God as we understood Him" (Covington, 1994, p. 43). Even with the wiggle room that "as we understood Him," seems to offer, the capital H-Him maintains the framework of the Christian God as a male deity. This step is among those that are so explicitly sexist and exclusionary that it will undoubtedly call for rhetorical acrobatics for Covington to make it woman-friendly.

In acknowledging that not only might the Christian God not work for every person in AA, but also that "turning one's will over to a man" is problematic for some women, Covington writes: "Women frequently say they fear everything will fall apart if they stop trying to control. But consider this instead: *it may be that things are supposed to fall apart*, and we'll only exhaust ourselves trying to prevent that from happening" (1994, p. 45). Rhetorically speaking, Covington's interpretation of the third step amounts to finding a synonym to the main point of the step. Where "submission" to God/Him "can be a special concern to us, because women are traditionally expected to yield to someone else's control," Covington offers "surrender" as an alternative way to think about submission, writing: "When we submit, we give in to a force that's trying to control us. When we surrender, we let go of our need to control" (1994, p. 48). This savvy reinterpretation turns a passive act into an active doing. Later in the chapter, the words "cooperate," "discovering our right to decide for ourselves," and "saying yes to life" all characterize surrendering in the sense of actively letting go of control as an act of self-love.

Covington's text reflects astute observations on the ways that AA is inherently sexist and deliberate attempts to reconcile the steps with women-centric frameworks. Mary Walker (2014) similarly acknowledged the well-known contradiction among many of the AA steps, from admitting one is powerless over their drinking to taking responsibility for one's actions. She noted that a way to bridge the gap between these poles is to rely on the concept of narrative, given that personal narrative is commonly used in AA meetings and writings. She writes that narratives are:

> used in bringing people into the program, describing progress, and making sense of experiences of addiction and recovery. The constant

exchange of personal stories within Twelve Step group practices provides templates for self-understanding to members, so that throughout
their recovery they may reinterpret themselves and their lives.

(Walker, 2014, p. 35)

In particular, Walker relies on Riceour's concept of "emplotment" (see also
Prussing, 2007), defining it as: "unifying discordant events into a whole,
combining diversity, variability, discontinuity, and instability into unities via
narrative" (2014, p. 35). Walker writes that this allows people to "interpret
their own lives within self-narratives that make their lives intelligible to them"
(2014, p. 35). She links this capacity of narrative to rectify the contradiction
between powerlessness and responsibility:

> If we can actively appropriate chance events into our identity by inter-
> preting them in terms of their role in our narrative, we could also actively
> appropriate actions over which we think of ourselves as powerless.
> Rather than being responsible only for free actions, we may assume
> responsibility for some action because we recognize that it plays a role
> in our identity; it is something that makes sense in light of other events
> [emplotted] in our narrative, and it contributes to the context that makes
> other events intelligible.
>
> (Walker, 2014, p. 37)

Therefore, in this logic, the discontinuity of "powerlessness" to "responsibility" is solved in the powerless actions' role in our identity formation—it may
be reconstituted into a narrative with its own logic—perhaps a then/now logic,
for instance.

As is evident, both practitioners and critics are interested in making
the discourse of AA make sense to audiences who question its logic, and
Covington's work is a worthwhile contribution to such efforts. While Walker
(2014) links the variability that narrative affords the individual to a semblance
of "its own logic," Covington embraces the contradictions to maintain the
power and helpfulness of this discourse for women: "there's something powerful and healing concealed beneath the archaic wording of the Steps. When
we look inside ourselves and reframe the original wording in the way that
worlds best for us, each of us, individually, can discover the meaning for
ourselves" (1994, p. 5).

While we do not hold AA any more accountable for its internal contradictions than any other person-made conceptual system to which adherents
flock to improve their lives, we do want to point out that the problems with
AA exceed many of the critiques of the program and have to do with its
stronghold in *doxa* as the main viable way to quit drinking and stay sober. In
the fraught cycles of patient epistemologies related to seeking sobriety, the
message that AA is the only or even best way can limit women's rhetorical

work and ultimately hurt their chances at a good outcome. Thus, we now turn to a text that offers a sobriety discourse less focused on convincing its audience that it works, and more focused on an original argument about alcoholism that seems to change the nature of the available frameworks for understanding one's alcoholism: Holly Whitaker's (2019) *Quit Like a Woman: The Radical Choice to Not Drink in a Culture Obsessed with Alcohol.*

Analysis of Quit Like a Woman, *2019 (QLAW)*

QLAW by Holly Whitaker is a more recent (2019) best-selling book that has dual purposes: to make a new argument about women's sobriety as a revolution against the "imperialistic white supremacist capitalist patriarchy" of bell hooks' description and to explain Whitaker's approach to becoming sober, which led to the founding of an online program called Tempest (2021, p. 20). Whitaker herself became sober in 2012 and has become well-known through her writing and social media presence. Rhetorically speaking, *QLAW* participates in the main feature of traditional sobriety discourse by sharing her personal story. However, the book is distinct in its use of researched information and statistics about alcohol and alcohol use disorder in the US, as well as the formation of a novel theory of sobriety:

> To properly heal from addiction [...] we need to address one of the bigger issues that women and other historically oppressed folks need to consider, which is how patriarchal structures affect the root causes of addiction, how they dominate the recovery landscape, and what that means for how we experience recovery.
>
> (Whitaker, 2021, p. 98)

Our analysis of this text focuses on its main claims about alcoholism and sobriety that question the traditional discourses and understandings and the dominance of AA, and that offer a new framework for meaning-making for women.

Whitaker situates her book in the specific moment of the #MeToo and Trump era in which women have taken to the streets and to social media to call out, disrupt, and protest systems of injustice. In that context, she says women are:

> Finally, *finally*, able to behold what a few millennia of patriarchy has done to us. We see and have words for the myriad ways racism, classism, sexism, homophobia [...] and endless systems of injustice, discrimination, and domination took root, and we are furiously working to dismantle all of it [...] What I want to know is why. Why are we so mad

at everything and not mad at what alcohol is doing to us, or how Big
Alcohol lines its pockets from our exploitation and death?

(2021, p. 38, emphasis in original)

Citing examples of death rates, alcohol use disorder, and sexual assault
involving alcohol, Whitaker provocatively argued that alcohol use disorder
is a result of women's oppression within the patriarchy and is made more
insipid by capitalism. Calling the alcohol industry "Big Alcohol" is a purposeful comparison to Big Tobacco, an industry whose harmful marketing
practices were eventually recognized and curbed mightily through legal
means. Whitaker compares drinking to smoking at length, arguing that not
only should drinking be negatively regarded in the same manner as smoking
has for a large segment of the US population, but that the American public
should be as critical of the alcohol industry as it has been of the tobacco
industry to reduce its harm (2021, p. 61). In particular, says Whitaker, the
marketing aimed at women is particularly ironic and dangerous. Whitaker
writes:

> It's hard not to draw parallels between the tobacco industry and the alco-
> hol industry when it comes to this type of marketing scheme [aimed at
> women]. Big Alcohol used the same liberated imagery and co-opted the
> same feminist ideals [i.e., drinking as independence], and women like
> me lapped it up.
>
> (2021, p. 57)

And, unlike smoking, people's conception of the problem of drinking is still
focused on the individual and not on the industry, as evidenced by the alcohol
industry's disclaimer "drink responsibly" (Whitaker, 2021, p. 61). Whitaker
argues there is a needed shift in identification and responsibility.

Whitaker's ideas may be taking hold. A 2021 study by Emily Nicholls
of 17 recently sober women's narratives revealed themes of identity in a
capitalist context, including the women describing their drinking selves as
counterproductive, reaching for "productivity" as a measure of a good neoliberal consumer (p. 774). Additionally, the women's turning point stories
lean heavily toward issues of identity, with the realization that one was far
beyond or beneath appropriate behaviors for an "enterprising and authen-
tic self" (Nicholls, 2021, p. 777). Nicholls questioned the influence of the
consumerist wellness culture of yoga, exercise, and "authenticity" on the
women, given that they replace drinking as culturally reinforced and encour-
aged consumer behavior with other consumer goods and services and especially those connected with wellness: "Participants actively reworked their
resistance [to drinking] in ways that still positioned them within dominant
consumer markets" (2021, p. 779). Still, Nicholls' study aligns with the suggestion that women may be choosing to resist drinking in part to resist the

alcohol-industrial complex, though still within a neoliberal understanding of the empowered self as consumer (2021, p. 778).

Whitaker also presents a claim about alcoholism itself, offering a two-part explanation after a review of the various definitions that have been used over time, including the choice theory, the self-medicating theory, the disease model, the learning model, and the dislocation model (2021, pp. 94–95). She asserts alcoholism is a "two-part problem" of root cause and "what happens to us […] over time when we use an effective but addictive substance or behavior in an attempt to regulate ourselves" (Whitaker, 2021, p. 98). In the disease view of alcoholism, the onus is on the individual needing to change, which aligns with the traditional AA discourse.

Carol Reeves (2019) explains how the theory of alcoholism as a disease emerged in the late 19th and early 20th century among practitioners who countered the prevailing ideas of addicts as moral failures or of bad character (p. 415). Reeves analyzed 92 medical papers published between 1870 and 1930, revealing that medical scholars and writers attempted to change perceptions and advance medical treatment for people in recovery not only through medical jargon, but also narratives, cultural tropes, and political language. Reeves found a "rich intermingling of scientific, literary, and political rhetorics" that "identifies humanizing narratives profiling special beings, ordinary citizens, and sympathetic others. Rather than a single theory of addiction as a disease of individuals, it reveals a significant emphasis on environmental factors" (2019, p. 439).

Kristen Cole and Anna Carmon (2019) additionally speak to the medicalization of addiction in addiction obituaries as a means of "help[ing] writers explain, in a concrete way, the physical and psychological effects of addiction in order to define it as a large-scale health crisis, as well as conveying it as a personal affliction or social problem" (p. 311). They remark that medicalization discourse of addiction is a "positive tool in many ways [though] one of its drawbacks is that it may serve to adapt people into existing social conditions rather than encouraging them to change these conditions" (Cole & Carmon, 2019, p. 315).

Whitaker neatly summarizes the structure of AA in order to suggest that it reinforces patriarchal limits on men who are outside the norm, which concurs with Travis' (2009) analysis noted above:

> The message of traditional recovery is that you need to shut up and listen. It says you need to go to ninety meetings in ninety days, adopt this label, know your place, read this book, work this program, do this thing. It says you don't know and you can't be trusted – the program is smarter than you are, all you have to do is work it and it will work.
>
> (Whitaker, 2021, p. 126)

Whitaker's reaction to the discourse was to recognize that as a woman already oppressed and internalizing societal expectations aimed at women all her life, she had to:

listen to [myself], and set out on my path [...] To finally heal, I didn't need to deny myself further, I needed to lift up the parts of me that had been forever repressed and denied. I also didn't need a map created by a man; I needed my own damn map.

(2021, p. 127)

The map metaphor interestingly relates to the procedure and guide that Whitaker craved—a way of understanding the problem and how she might solve it differently than had been offered through the traditional sobriety discourses.

This text shows a marked change over the course of time in the available discourses of sobriety for women resulting from multiplied and increasing voices, particularly through women-focused studies and perhaps with a nod to the usefulness of social media, although a true understanding of its impact in an evidence-based manner is outside the scope of this book. Still, within this change, we observe an expansion of rhetorical possibilities and with them, epistemologies—the meaning-making opportunities for women to grapple with the health flashpoint of seeking sobriety.

Outdated and inadequate: Jamie's rhetorical encounters at the health flashpoint of seeking sobriety

My (Jamie's) "sobriety journey," a metaphor often used for many health and medical treatments, began with a tumult of three overlapping and disorienting discourses on a single morning, the day of my diagnosis as a moderate alcoholic in March 2018. This "rhetorical encounter"—or series of them—along with my reactions to them, with time, ultimately revealed themselves to be an interesting example of a very intense early rhetorical encounter that immediately shaped my perceptions of what was happening and the rhetorical community of sobriety I was about to enter into—even if, on that day, these discourses were simultaneously helpful, humbling, confusing, insulting, and infuriating.

The encounters began with medical discourse in my general practitioner's exam room when she used the DSM 5 to assess and diagnose me with moderate alcoholism. She immediately suggested I take a leave of absence from work to seek treatment and began preparing Family Medical Leave Act paperwork. Walking out to my car, I was shocked and dazed but proceeded to the HR office at work, where my colleagues immediately reacted to my doctor's paperwork and began to speak the language of bureaucracy, explaining the FMLA and our Employee Assistance Program, focusing on my benefits package and how many hours my leave would entail. I was overwhelmed, but grateful. These medical and bureaucratic discourses came on suddenly, and I was surprised to find myself the subject of these words, but I appreciated that the doctor and my HR colleagues were clinical yet kind in their delivery, their main interests being to help me and do their procedures correctly.

In contrast, the last stop of the morning is where I encountered the more well-known and loaded dominant narrative of sobriety, enacted by a supervisor at work whose inappropriate reaction to my disclosure cleaved exactly to male-centric understandings of alcoholism based on assumptions about age, class, and hitting "rock bottom." This supervisor was otherwise an educated and caring person, evidencing the cultural power of stock narratives about alcoholism, and the prevalence of anti-support we have identified in our study with breast cancer patients—well-meaning, but ultimately hurtful.

I acknowledge my very lucky and privileged circumstances that allowed me to have a private professional addiction counselor, health insurance that paid for some of that treatment, partially-paid time off from work, and a supportive and caring network of people in my life. As a teacher, I also had an entire summer to "do the work" before returning to work the next fall. However, in pursuing examples of how to "do sobriety" outside of AA, I felt a little like an outsider, or like someone who was forging a new path—or, perhaps more accurately, a hidden path since many middle-class people like me who avail themselves of similar treatment options might not "go public" with their process. On the path I chose, there was a sense that what I was doing was singular, shameful, and not meant for middle-aged moms who work at universities.

Note that, even in private, professional addiction treatment, the discourse of AA is an influential force; my counselor used the Covington interpretation of the twelve steps in my treatment plan. This offers further evidence that this amateur, culturally-approved self-help discourse has been adopted by professionals and dominates the world of sobriety. Despite my initial perception that a lack of alternatives existed, I found *Hip Sobriety*, which alerted me to the fact that alternative discourses for sobriety particularly around women's experiences have at least started to expand, becoming more visible on the internet, in published memoirs, and in self-help books with *QLAW* exemplifying these changes.

Expanding rhetorics, Expanding epistemologies

Throughout this chapter, we have presented the ways that scholars and practitioners have considered the traditional and potentially radical rhetorics of/ and women's sobriety. By way of conclusion, we wish to call attention to the potential hegemonic implications of uncritically accepting dominant discourses as the only or best way to understand and/or do sobriety or make meaning during any health circumstance. In our study of the types of support that helped or hurt women breast cancer patients, we learned that some well-established and accepted comments, arguments, or frameworks for understanding breast cancer patients' experiences can cause more harm than help. In Chapter 4, we established that repeated messages about women and menopause stagnate activism. Jamie's sobriety experience suggests the same.

Therefore, we suggest additional rhetorical options within sobriety discourse besides narrative that can help to make meaning of one's situation and identity as a sober person to diversify rhetorical encounters, expand understanding, and improve support. Such alternatives should also posit non-AA ways of getting and staying sober.

Metaphors

In our analysis of Covington's (1994) text above, we noted the main metaphors at play including the lotus flower and the development of babies. Jamie also found a commonly used grief metaphor helpful in her recovery. This is the metaphor of grief being a hole that you are stepping gingerly around with no space. The hole is the grief, and it has your attention all the time at first because it is gaping in your space and has a dangerous, cliff-edge feel to it. Eventually, while the hole does not shrink, the space around it expands as your life continues. You learn to live right near the grief but have the option to step back and make use of the additional space around it. You can regard the hole from some distance or get close up to it sometimes, which is painful, but it is not all-consuming the way it is early on in recovery/fresh grief. We caution the support person to be wary of the uncritical metaphor such as "warrior" as is common in breast cancer rhetoric, or "rock bottom" as is common in sobriety discourse.

Dissoi logoi

Whitaker (2021) acknowledges the contradictions inherent in sobriety work when she references an adage by Pema Chodron to be both big and small at the same time: "big, as in we are worthy because we exist. Small, as in we exist to serve humanity. Such is the extension we navigate when coming at recovery with a culturally inflicted deficit of self-worth" (p. 140). This speaks to finding ways other than "narrative" to explain things to yourself or understand what it is you're doing. In rhetorical terms, we might name it *dissoi logoi*, or a "method of intellectual exploration" that allows for the abstract definition of a word or concept to co-exist with a specific instance (Bizzell and Herzberg, p. 47). In this way, the rhetorical action of *dissoi logoi* or contextualizing contradictions in sobriety work may "destabilize the unquestioned authority of arguments based on essential qualities," the assumed essential qualities of alcoholism having been duly noted in the literature and subjects of analysis in this chapters (p. 47).

In my (Jamie's) experience, I made meaning by learning to accept contradictions and actually resisting the creation of a cohesive narrative since that seemed to me like "explaining things away" too easily. In my case, I needed to state true facts about my life which were incongruous, an act which was more helpful than telling my life story in a neat narrative. For me, embracing contradictions meant acknowledging (with some difficulty and pain) that my life had elements of pain based on some early trauma that probably contributed to addiction, but that fact did not negate the positive people and experiences in my life as well. Both things are true, and simply getting clear that a condition of contraries could exist was a very helpful epistemological project.

Embracing more definitions of alcoholism and sobriety

Alongside the dominant definition of alcoholism and assumptions about what sobriety entails, there are a growing number of different understandings of alcoholism and sobriety, especially on social media where one might discover movements or affinity groups such as The New Sobriety, the term Sober-Curious, "going damp," and the advent of Dry January. Jamie's preferred term for her moderate alcoholism, for instance, is "alcoholish." These movements emphasize, as does Whitaker, that not drinking is a choice that can be difficult in a society "obsessed with alcohol" but one that can provide benefits, even if one does not identify in the traditional manner as a full-blown alcoholic (meaning, "rock bottom" public male with a DUI for example). These movements have been criticized for bringing the idea of "choice" into sobriety, given that some with alcohol abuse disorders may have little choice beyond life or death because of their addictions (see, for an example of this critique, Dresner, 2020). Amy Dresner also points out that the "Straight Edge" movement far predates the radical notion of *QLAW*. Nicholls (2021) might also critique these movements' emphasis on self-care practices as trends driven by consumerism and marketing. That said, we argue and believe that the field of rhetorical studies would endorse a position that "more is more" when it comes to ways of understanding that will help more people name their experiences and empower themselves. A monolithic framework with AA at the center, we contend, limits more than it encourages a diversity of patients' cycles of epistemologies.

Embracing Whitaker's two-pronged definition of alcoholism is one option, as well as embracing the "grey area" that the New Sobriety represents when it comes to problematic drinking or alcohol use disorder. These definitions have two consequences: first, they afford whomever feels disenfranchised from the dominant AA discourse a conception of themselves and a way forward into sobriety. Second, the afforded identifications by each new individual in turn creates a more diverse conception of alcoholism and sobriety societally, which will iterate and grow, allowing more identifications and more conceptions as "alcoholic" becomes less and less confined to the dominant definition and "sobriety" becomes less and less confined to the dominant discourses.

Prussing's (2007) study shows that, for instance, younger women do not want or need the traditional rubric of alcoholism and do not harken back to a time "before" alcohol made the impression it did in their lives because, in many native women's case, there is no "before" alcohol entered their lives and family. Instead these women shaped their own definitions by living their own values, rather than being drawn "back" to a traditional time when their ancestors were considered more noble or pure, which Prussing refers to as the rhetoric of the empty center (p. 499).

Resisting assumptions and asking questions

The critique of the dominant and adoption of lesser, co-existing discourses of sobriety is growing, and these shifts will help not only those seeking sobriety but also their support people in using language differently to proliferate the conceptions we track above. Such things could help the sobriety-seeker in positive and affirming ways, especially through resisting *doxastic* understandings of alcoholism and sobriety. More work can be done to open space for new types of questions that dominant assumptions preempt. For example, support persons might consider new questions around.

Treatment

It may behoove sobriety-seekers if their support people do not assume they will attend AA and instead ask: how are you pursuing treatment? We learned from our breast cancer study that offers of rides and company during first treatment sessions or particularly stressful or scary appointments is often a welcome support.

Counting days

The AA habit of counting days, weeks, months, and years and giving and receiving tokens for periods of sobriety is unappealing if a sobriety-seeker is not able to live a perfect "before and after" narrative of their journey. Pekka Lund (2016) found that multiple attempts at sobriety were common in her study of paths to sobriety. Support people can avoid asking about time if that information is not offered and instead ask what health or life changes the sobriety-seeker has been experiencing.

Mocktails and dry events

Questions will lead the way here for support people; simply ask what the sobriety-seeker would prefer at events where control of the drink menu is possible.

The discourses surrounding women's ways of doing sobriety would seem to suggest that there are many viable alternatives to Christian-centric, male-dominated, and heteronormative AA discourses, but the rhetorical framework of AA is always residually present, even in the professional sphere. We have identified the difficulty for the individual to seek an individual path forward. The aim of this chapter has been to show how and why alternatives lend themselves to stronger cycles of patient epistemologies when women seek sobriety.

References

Anderson, C. M., & MacCurdy, M. (2000). *Writing & healing: Toward an informed practice*. NCTE.

Bizzell, P., & Herzberg, B. (Eds.). (1990). *The rhetorical tradition: Readings from classical times to the present*. St. Martin's Press.

Cole, K. L., & Carmon, A. F. (2019). Changing the face of the opioid epidemic: A generic rhetorical analysis of addiction obituaries. *Rhetoric of Health & Medicine, 2*(3), 291–320. https://doi.org/10.5744/rhm.2019.1014

Covington, S. S. (1994). *A woman's way through the twelve steps*. Hazelden Publishing.

Dowsett-Johnston, A. (2014). *Drink: The intimate relationship between women and alcohol*. Harper.

Dresner, A. (2020, January 27). The "New Sobriety:" Can it be both a health trend and a matter of life and death? *Psychology Today*. https://www.psychologytoday.com/us/blog/coming-clean/202001/the-new-sobriety

Hogg, E. J. (2019). After alcohol: Gender and sobriety counterstories in two contemporary novels. *The Social History of Alcohol. and Drugs, 33*(2), 310–335. https://doi.org/10.1086/705338

Lund, P. (2016). Christianity in narratives of recovery from substance abuse. *Pastoral Psychology, 65*(3), 351–368. https://doi.org/10.1007/s11089-016-0687-3

Nicholls, E. (2021). Sober rebels or good consumer-citizens? Anti-consumption and the 'enterprising self' in early sobriety. *Sociology, 55*(4), 768–784. https://doi.org/10.1177/0038038520981837

Pennebaker, J. (1990). *Opening up: The healing power of expressing emotions*. Guilford.

Prussing, E. (2007). Reconfiguring the empty center: Drinking, sobriety, and identity in Native American women's narratives. *Culture, Medicine and Psychiatry, 31*(4), 499–526. https://doi.org/10.1007/s11013-007-9064-0

Reeves, C. (2019). Medical rhetoric and the sympathetic "inebriet": 1870–1930. *Rhetoric of Health & Medicine, 2*(4), 415–445. https://doi.org/10.5744/rhm.2019.1019

Ryan, K. J. (2010). Making pathways: Inventing textual research methods in feminist rhetorical studies. In E. E. Schell & K. J. Rawson (Eds.), *Rhetorica in motion: Feminist rhetorical methods and methodologies* (pp. 89–103). University of Pittsburgh Press.

Travis, T. (2009). "Handles to hang on to our sobriety": Commonplace books and surrendered masculinity in Alcoholics Anonymous. *Men and Masculinities, 12*(2), 175–200. https://doi.org/10.1177/1097184X08318182

Walker, M. J. (2014). Powerlessness and responsibility in twelve step narratives. In J. Miller & N. Plants (Eds.), *Sobering wisdom: Philosophical explorations of twelve step spirituality* (pp. 30–41). University of Virginia Press.

Whitaker, H. (2021). *Quit like a woman: The radical choice to not drink in a culture obsessed with alcohol.* Random House Publishing Group.

6 A rhetorical autoethnographic sketch of patient epistemology

For the last 19 years, I (Bryna) have been writing about cancer, specifically breast cancer but sometimes just cancer in general, and how it has affected my life and the lives of my family members. When I learned that I am BRCA2+, meaning I have a mutation in my BRCA2 gene that makes me susceptible to breast, ovarian, pancreatic, and other types of cancer, in many ways cancer became the focus of my life, even though I didn't actually develop cancer until several years later.

Having a genetic mutation means I inherited this susceptibility from a parent, in my case from my father, who inherited it from his own father, whose sisters also most likely had it, considering they both died from breast and/or ovarian cancer. My grandfather's mother, who suffered from ovarian cancer, also probably had the gene mutation, as do many of my cousins, several of whom have survived various types of cancer (breast, lung, skin).

For a long time now, I've been writing about all of us, but mostly about my own experiences with cancer, and in several ways: My blog, *Blogging BRCA: The BRCA Experience in Real Time*, which I started in December 2012 and was, for several years, linked to a national cancer support organization's website; in public writing in the form of blog posts for the *Philadelphia Inquirer's* "Diagnosis: Cancer" series; in Facebook posts to friends and family who had joined my group, "Bryna's BC Updates;" a small handful of articles published in academic journals; and privately, in a folder on my computer called "BRCA Book," which contains various vignettes from me and some of my cousins, as we always hoped to put together a multi-genre book about our family; and in random Word documents stored in a folder called, "Breast Cancer Creative Writing."

The present book, which is overall about finding support and making meaning from women's health and medical embodied experiences, asks epistemological questions about how women come to understand those experiences, experiences such as mine, and the sources of support that come along with them. In this chapter, I aim to craft a rhetorical autoethnography that offers ways to understand and acknowledge how a patient comes to understand her identity as a patient. My methods of analysis and constructing a rhetorical autoethnography are taken in part from Brett Lunceford (2015) who explains:

DOI: 10.4324/9781003398318-6

We already tell stories within criticism. Any engaging work will involve a clear discussion of the context of the rhetoric in question, and this often takes the form of narrative exposition. The reader is able to "see" the work as it happened.

(p. 7)

He continues:

There is a difference between caring about an issue and caring about a person. This is precisely what autoethnography does—it reminds us that the individuals we write about are actually living, breathing human beings.

(p. 8)

Thus, this chapter seeks to portray a living, breathing human's health experience through a critical and rhetorical context. My methods follow Kim Hensley Owens (2019), whose rhetorical autoethnography, "Writing My Body, Writing My Health," describes over twenty years of writing about her own health. Like Hensley Owens, my goal is to "let readers connect to me as both a writer and as an embodied being," while also "explor[ing] the functions, forms, and value of various examples of my writing" (p. 15). I aim to enhance "understandings of disparate rhetorical artifacts"—my own writings, as listed above—and "make rhetorical sense...of my own health-related personal and public writing" (p. 15). Lastly, I use "analytical vignettes" as Hensley Owens does (p. 15)—short excerpts from my own writing along with brief rhetorical analysis.

More specifically, in this chapter I use the rhetorical concept of *aporia* to analyze my own writing. As discussed in Chapter 3, *aporia* or absurdity became obvious within our data as a way to understand contradictory or confusing sets of truths during women's breast cancer experiences. According to Stuart Murray (2009), "If we arrive at an aporia, it means we are in doubt, we are perplexed, we are confused about how (best) to proceed. There is seemingly no exit, an intrinsic undecidability. An aporia is a contradiction, a puzzle or a paradox" (p. 11).

Feeling aporetic is the result of an absurd proposition, a proposition outside the bounds of human reason. In fact, writing this at all might be aporetic: illogical, absurd, and contradictory. At the time of this writing, the world is suffering through a global pandemic. The scale of "worst thing that can happen" to a person has shifted as, at the time of this writing, almost seven million people have died from COVID-19 worldwide.

Before the pandemic, most people would arguably have agreed that one of the worst things that could happen to them would be a cancer diagnosis; for a woman, a breast cancer diagnosis might be the worst thing that happens in her life. I can say with some authority (and perhaps melodrama) that when one is diagnosed with cancer, one has a lot of existential questions: why me? Why is my life of so little value that I've been chosen to suffer the surgeries, the treatments, and the various horrors that are cancer in the modern day? These answers are never revealed unless perhaps one subscribes to an organized religion in which a deity helps locate them. But there are epistemological questions as well—how do I come to understand what's going on in my body, what's being done to me by my medical team, and how I'm being treated by friends and loved ones? How do I make meaning from this, and/or make this meaningful? This is where rhetorical autoethnography comes in.

Some background

After living with the knowledge of my BRCA2 mutation for almost seven years, I decided I couldn't take the constant anxiety of wondering when, not if, I would develop cancer. So, I began interviewing surgeons to perform a prophylactic oophorectomy (removal of the ovaries), full hysterectomy (removal of the uterus, fallopian tubes, and cervix), and mastectomy (removal of the breasts). Removal, removal, removal: a slightly less aggressive word than "amputation," nonetheless a seemingly archaic way of solving any problem in the body, yet considered the best course of action for preventing cancer when one has mutated BRCA genes. That anxiety leads to a false sense of choice; as Kelly Pender (2018) explains, "rhetorics of choice have allowed those at genetic risk to believe that they have freely chosen what they were, in fact, compelled to choose" (p. 1).

During this time, I began writing my blog. Initially, I did this so that I had a place to keep my notes from all of the doctor's appointments. I made it public, however, because there was, at the time, so little information and writing about BRCA that I felt an obligation to the BRCA community to track my experiences so that others like me could learn what it was like. In this way, I sought to fulfill a "'rhetorical need,' a need that is fulfilled (1) only in writing, (2) for a specific audience, and (3) for the purposes of engaging that audience rhetorically (to act)" (Siegel Finer, 2016, p. 177). Previvors, or those with a genetic predisposition to cancer, fulfill specific rhetorical needs when they blog, which include educating others, advocating for research and funding into BRCA and breast cancer, and supporting their community (p. 177).

While I was interviewing surgeons, I faced an unexpected turn of events. During a routine mammogram (mammograms for BRCA+ people are routine even if the person is not the recommended age of 40+), I was diagnosed with Ductal Carcinoma in Situ (DCIS) in my right breast. DCIS is considered pre-cancer or Stage 0 cancer, but with a genetic mutation, it is taken as seriously as cancer, and my prophylactic surgeries were no longer considered optional (or preventative). Within a month, I had a double mastectomy with flap reconstruction (abdominal fat and muscle removed and then used to reconstruct breasts); five months later, I had the hysterectomy/oophorectomy, and another five months later, I had a revision to the original breast surgery. At my year-out checkup from the mastectomy, I was considered cancer-free, cured, no evidence of disease (NED). I went for check-ups annually to have my reconstructed breasts professionally palpated, and for five years, everything seemed to be fine.

Five years after I was diagnosed with DCIS, I wrote about my experience for Philly.com's Diagnosis Cancer column:

> The physician's assistant keeps saying how great it is to celebrate five years cancer-free with me. I don't feel nearly as excited about this as she does. I realize I don't want to be free. I have reduced my cancer risk as much as a BRCA-positive woman can – having a double-mastectomy, removing my ovaries, then having a total hysterectomy to eliminate any space for cancer. But I know there is only risk reduction, never risk elimination.
>
> (Siegel Finer, 2018)

Here, I am identifying a clear disjunction between the mood of the PA and my own. The mood of the PA seems reasonably positive—her patient is cured—and my own would probably be considered pessimistic. Still, I knew the need for continued vigilance.

Exactly six months later, I found a lump on the side of my right reconstructed breast while soaping my underarm in the shower. As in so many movies, I stopped and stood with water running over my head until it turned cold, with my fingers pressed against this lump. I tried to remember what we're all told about breast lumps—round good, misshapen bad; moveable good, stuck in place bad. Mine felt round and moveable—good—though I hardly trusted myself with this amateur diagnosis; I somehow knew without a doubt that some of the pre-cancerous cells that were "removed" so many years earlier had been left behind and had turned hard, angry, malignant. My surgeon's PA squeezed me into her schedule that afternoon. Within a few weeks, I'd had a biopsy, an appointment with the surgeon, a trip planned to Philadelphia for a consultation with the nation's top BRCA researcher/doctor, and surgery scheduled. I was diagnosed with invasive ductal carcinoma (IDC), Stage 2A, treatable with surgery, chemotherapy, and radiation. It hadn't spread outside of my breast. I was supposed to consider myself lucky.

But I didn't. I was far from grateful—I was furious. Furious at my doctors, who I (erroneously) suspected hadn't done all they could have in those years before (misplaced blame), but mostly furious at myself for having been fooled all those years. What about the surgeries I'd spent a year undergoing and recovering from six years earlier? Had those been a total waste of time, energy, and money? What had I done to myself in those intervening years that contributed to this development? Ate too much ice cream. Exercised not nearly enough. Why hadn't I sought a second opinion back then? Did I really know enough about that situation that I should have accepted my doctors' prognosis—cured—even when I knew my DNA was bad?

To deal with my anger and separate myself from the diagnosis, I turned my cancer into an academic project. I scoured over all my doctors' notes from when I'd had DCIS and the current round of information as it came in. I became a near-expert on reading pathology reports, the queen of Google, a pubMed ninja, and I published all of my findings on my blog. I planned never to be surprised again, and I wasn't. I knew everything I needed to know always before stepping into a doctor's office. Doing academic-type research on my diagnosis helped me not only to learn more about what was going on in my body but also helped me to take ownership of it. While spending endless days waiting to hear from doctors with test results, I could, by using information I already had, predict what those results would show. I wasn't at the mercy of time. I had wrested some control over a fate and a set of genetic circumstances that felt, frankly, so far out of my control.

Throughout recovery from surgery and many months of treatment, I was supported by family, friends, and colleagues in many ways. It is amazing what a cancer diagnosis can do to your sense of independence. Even if you think you can do something on your own, someone is there offering to do it for you. This was a double-edged sword for me—ever Type A—having the aporic effect of making me feel supported, yet also making me feel like no one thought I could do things myself. It was something I never wrote about, even in my private documents, because the idea that I might be ungrateful for the support, and not the cancer patient from the standard narrative, was too hard to understand or acknowledge.

For instance, a lasagna left at the front door would make me feel sad, but a bitmoji of us drinking margaritas sent from a friend over text would make me gleeful. A gift bag with fuzzy socks and a novel was delightful, but a request for information to help set up a meal train felt overwhelming. I wrote thank you notes to every last person who sent something from afar or dropped something off at our house—whether food, comfort items, no matter how sick I felt—everyone received a thank you note. Perhaps that is why some of the support felt burdensome; I burdened myself.

As we describe in Chapter 2, the process of developing a patient epistemology, or, understanding one's own identity as a patient, takes place in a series of often repeating steps: health flashpoint, rhetorical encounters, decision-making, and reflection/reshaping/recapitulating. These steps can take place over time or in one instance, as shown here, in my blog entry from July 11, 2019:

> This morning, my husband and I met with Dr. McAuliffe to find out prognosis and treatment plan. The cancer is stage 2A (not terrible; totally treatable). After looking at scans and pathology from 2013, she is pretty certain that this is the same cancer (just as I suspected) I had then – as

many DCIS cells as possible were removed during my mastectomy. But the doctors always said they can never remove every single cell. I like to make this analogy – it's like a carton of ice cream. Even after you scoop out all of the ice cream, there's still a little bit of ice cream residue that remains in the carton. Same thing here – they made a cut in the bottom of my breast, scooped out all of the breast tissue, but there was always going to be a little bit of residual tissue remaining. The chances of that tissue becoming cancerous are practically nil, but hey, they took a chance on me and won the jackpot! It only takes one rogue mother fucker; this one hung around, grew, and now it's invasive and is spreading throughout my breast. I suppose, luckily, I felt it before it did too much damage; it is not in my lymph nodes or elsewhere in my body. Still, we are going to treat it aggressively because I am not going through this a third time.

(Siegel Finer, 2019)

I continue later in this same blog post:

Some ask me how I'm feeling about all of this, and to be honest, I don't feel anything. I did feel pretty nervous this morning before the appointment, but Dr. McAuliffe was so caring and thorough, and I think my preliminary research helped me see this as an academic enterprise and keep some emotional distance from it. I diagnosed myself after all – no huge surprises in the exam room today.

(Siegel Finer, 2019)

In this post, I see myself grappling with my diagnosis, "the cancer" and not "my cancer," the health flashpoint I experienced in Dr. McAuliffe's office, moving through that moment into a rhetorical encounter with some preliminary research I'd done based on my pathology reports. I go through some rhetorical work of decision-making (agreeing to treat aggressively so that it does not return) and then arrive at some reflection (how do I feel about all of this?). While the process is not necessarily linear (in fact, in this example, it's rather simultaneous), each step represents some encounter with language that helps me to process or understand my identity as a person with cancer. In the end, I understand my diagnosis ("no surprises in the exam room today"), although I don't necessarily accept it or interpolate it into my identity as such.

Below, I go into more depth and rhetorically analyze these four steps toward a patient epistemology as they appear throughout my private and public writing.

Flashpoint

As I said above, when I learned that I had invasive cancer, I was angry. Mostly I was angry at myself, feeling that I hadn't been vigilant enough with my health in order to keep cancer at bay. I also became angry with my everyday life. Having cancer became a full-time job. A doctor's office would call and tell me that I had an appointment for a test or a scan or a blood draw or a consultation; no one asked what my calendar looked like or if I was available to do these things. I recognized the privilege of being on summer break from my teaching position, and I was grateful that my son had camp to go to each day, so I was "available;" yet I had hoped to do research and writing that summer, not spend it driving to and from the hospital. Nevertheless, that's what I did, and I became frustrated and resentful that my summer was sucked away by cancer. Everywhere I turned, it seemed like someone was demanding something of my time, and the minutiae of daily life took its toll.

On July 2, 2019, almost one month to the day that I was diagnosed with invasive breast cancer, while awaiting to learn of my surgery date, I wrote the following on my personal blog:

> Even when you know that cancer is growing in your body, even when you can feel the lump every time you put on your bra or wash under your arm in the shower, life continues to go on. Your alarm goes off in the morning and you get out of bed. You continue to put laundry in the washing machine, to feed the dog, to go through all the minutiae of life. You call Comcast to negotiate a better deal when your Wi-Fi bill suddenly goes up $30 a month, and when they won't cave, you cancel it and sign up for Verizon. You order four pairs of sneakers for your son, and when they arrive, you have him try them all on, choose one that fits right, then package them all up again to take to the UPS store. You go to the library to pick up and return books. You do the weed whacking around the fence where the lawn mower doesn't quite reach and the grass grows so high it begins to look like a meadow. You do all of these things even if you don't know how bad your cancer is, if you should be using your time more wisely, savoring every minute, making a bucket list, watching and memorizing every move your child makes. You start to wonder, as you crawl along the kitchen floor spraying Raid at an ant infestation, "I have cancer; shouldn't someone else do this?" and when you get an email that your homeowners insurance company is going to cancel if you don't cut some branches from a tree overhanging your roof, you think, "but I have cancer; isn't all forgiven for me?" And then you spend an hour looking for your property deed, searching online for the land survey that shows you don't own that tree, and emailing the realtor who sold you your house. Because shit just goes on, and someone has to do it, and no one really gives a flying fuck if you have cancer when you're the one who pays the bills.
>
> (Siegel Finer, 2019)

A flashpoint can be both acute and chronic, and here my writing shows how acute flashpoints contribute to meaning-making. Almost every day, a phone call or appointment would force me to relive my diagnosis and to live it out, snapping me out of the usual banality of my day to remind me that I had cancer. Additionally, each moment of that usual banality was a flashpoint, reminding me over and over of my diagnosis as those banalities became more challenging. Virginia Woolf (1926) writes, in *On Being Ill*:

> I am in bed with influenza—but what does that convey of the great experience; how the world has changed its shape; the tools of business grown remote; the sounds of festival become romantic like a merry-go-round heard across far fields... while the whole landscape of life lies remote and fair.
>
> (pp. 34–35)

No, all is not forgiven of me, just like it's not forgiven of anyone else who has experienced illness, which Woolf likens to a minor blip in the scenery of the "whole landscape of life." This is what makes the idea—that life should be forgiven when one has cancer—absurd: that others have suffered before me and will suffer after me. Yet, there is a disjunction here, in the way that my life has been taken over by cancer, yet Woolf is saying that illness conveys nothing about "the great experience" that is life.

Although absurd, or perhaps because of the absurd, my writing does at times subvert the agnotological narrative about cancer, demonstrating frustration and anger with no sense of comedy or talk of being "cured." This is not a survivor story; it is a "cry out, desperate, clamorously, for the divine relief of sympathy" (Woolf, 1926, p. 35). I am asking that the world take some pity on me and cease with all the mundane banalities of life because doing both (cancer and life) is too exhausting. This is absurdism in its classic form: "the tension which emerges from the individual's determination to discover purpose and order in a world which steadfastly refuses to evidence either" (Childs & Fowler, 2006, p. 1). This is most evident in the line, "you do all of these things even if you don't know how bad your cancer is, if you should be using your time more wisely, savoring every minute, making a bucket list, watching and memorizing every move your child makes" where I question how one can be expected to continue with everyday life when there are more important things to attend to. This presents a tension that "the world" is not going to allow me to negotiate—have cancer *and* attend to the banalities of daily life. There is no choice. I had to live in alternate universes simultaneously which is, of course, impossible, or, utterly absurd.

Rhetorical encounters

Almost immediately after diagnosis, I became an expert at researching and interpreting my own cancer documentation. Only a week after learning I had cancer, for example, I wrote on my blog:

I am a teacher and scholar of the way writing is used to make things happen. Of everything I learned in my education, what helps me the most in the real world is not my writing skills but my research skills. Not only am I adept at finding research, but I know how to read it, analyze it, critique it, and corroborate it.

(Siegel Finer, 2019)

As an English professor with a PhD in rhetoric and composition, I am fortunate to have strong research skills, familiarity with and access to health databases like CINHAL and PubMed, and time to read and analyze what I read. I spent nearly all of the time that I wasn't at doctor's appointments on the computer, searching for answers that I was too impatient to wait for from my doctors. Here, at the end of June 2019, I work hard to stage my own cancer:

In this PDF, I've copied Komen's chart and shaded in spaces that match up with my current diagnosis. Much depends on the first column; I know T2 because my tumor size is more than 2cm but less than 5cm (although a lot of the information I have found on where a 2cm tumor would be staged is contradictory – some would stage it as 1; some would stage it as 2); but I don't know node involvement or metastasis. Based on everything else I know, I think I'm looking at stage 1B, 2A, or 2B. Because the PET scan seemed to be clear (according to the tech in the room), I am going to assume no lymph involvement or metastasis, so my guess is that my cancer is stage 1B.

(Siegel Finer, 2019)

Knowing one's cancer stage allows one to know if chemotherapy will be a likely recommendation, so I was very anxious about where my cancer would be staged. While I didn't know all of the factors, I was able to determine an approximate cancer stage by working with information from my pathology reports and various scans. My writing in this post demonstrates three rhetorical encounters, or encounters with three discourses—one, the Komen chart; two, the exchange with the PET scan tech; and three, my pathology report. All contributed to my ability to understand my identity as a patient. Yet, of course, I couldn't know everything necessary to truly stage myself, not being an oncologist, relying on scraps of information that I didn't truly know how to put together.

Six months after my diagnosis, I began a funded sabbatical—a leave from my university work; until the COVID-19 pandemic began in earnest in the US in March 2020, I had two months of time to turn my cancer into an academic pursuit (time I should've been spending writing and working on academic research projects). I wrote in my blog in December 2019:

I'm on sabbatical now. So, as a fun side project, I will use the information presented in this secondary article and its primary research to predict whether my cancer is going to come back, despite the chemotherapy I am 3/4 of the way completed and the radiation therapy I will begin at the end of January. I am particularly interested in what my MRI reports say about tumor heterogeneity, and if there is research out there related to BRCA tumors and heterogeneity.

(Siegel Finer, 2019)

Reading this, one might think that the phrase, "as a fun side project" was tongue in cheek, and while I think it may have been at the time, looking back on it, I know that it was instead a survival strategy. Turning my own illness into an academic project, despite how absurd that might sound, provided me with an epistemological way to understand my own cancer, by participating in the discourse community in which I am so comfortable. While I could've learned about my cancer from the various pamphlets (indeed, a binder full of them) from my doctor, I instead sought out texts from researchers like myself who do empirical studies and present evidence from data without flourish. Through these rhetorical encounters, I reconciled a part of my identity—an academic researcher—with the new identity with which I was grappling—as a BRCA+ patient who, despite extreme prophylactic measures, was unlucky enough to get cancer anyway.

Rhetorical work

As we've discussed, oftentimes decision-making occurs when one is deciding whether to participate in the standard or stock narrative about an illness in order to make meaning from it.

Judy Segal (2008), as previously noted, demonstrates how this entrenched standard makes it nearly impossible to speak about breast cancer in any other way. If you write a narrative in which breast cancer sucks, or the end is that someone is miserable and sick, or you critique your doctors or the options available to women suffering from breast cancer—if you try to be an activist within the genre of "breast cancer narrative"—then you are bitter and maybe even said to be contributing to your own demise, as Barbara Ehrenreich's (2009) book *Bright-Sided* compellingly charts. In her aptly named chapter, "Smile or Die: The Bright Side of Cancer," Ehrenreich speaks out against the "tyranny of positive thinking" (p. 42), noting that "Positive thinking seems to be mandatory in the breast cancer world, to the point that unhappiness requires a kind of apology" (p. 26). She continues, "the sugar-coating of can-cer can exact a dreadful cost…[requiring] the denial of understandable feel-ings of anger and fear, all of which must be buried under a cosmetic layer of cheer" (p. 41). Despite how necessary it is to speak one's angry or fearful truth, in the case of accepted discourse around breast cancer, one who does so has not conformed to the genre, and so their narrative is dismissed. No one wants to read that. And therefore, the dialogue about breast cancer is never really advanced (p. 18). Segal refers to this as agnotological, or, perpetuating ignorance.

In some ways, my writing falls into the agnotological; in other ways, I subvert the typical narrative. In this blog entry, I do both:

> A lot of people in the BRCA community talk about the (not) choice between surveillance and surgery. Do you want your life to be run by a constant schedule of MRIs and mammograms required to surveil, or screen for, cancer when you are high risk, or do you want to have preventative surgery and, presumably, never go through one of those scans again? That decision was mostly made for me back in 2013 when pathologists found DCIS in my right breast, and I (not) chose to have a mastectomy to reduce the amount of breast tissue I had to practically nothing so as to avoid the chance of recurrence (of course, I had a recurrence anyway), and thus the need for surveillance (I also had a hysterectomy and my ovaries removed so as to eliminate the need to surveil anything "down there"). But, that (not) choice did effectively reduce my surveillance schedule to basically nothing.
>
> (Siegel Finer, 2020)

This excerpt simultaneously reproduces and subverts the standard narrative. In the writing, I use the word "(not)" in parenthesis as a way to demonstrate that these choices aren't really choices; I was, as Pender (2018) says, "neither in control nor ever really free to choose" (p. 1). By making the choices that are mostly made for us, one is participating in the standard narrative. By acknowledging it's not a choice, one can subvert that narrative. Both offer epistemological consequences as they helped me to make meaning from the standard discourse—I could participate in order to feel camaraderie, but (not) participate in order to feel empowered.

Absurdity figures into this sample, as well—absurdity as an impasse where one is asked to make a choice but the two options one is choosing between aren't really on even playing ground, or the "correct" choice is assumed. From a meaning-making standpoint, one must wonder why they are asked to make a choice at all.

Material and constitutive effects

Throughout my treatment, I suffered side effects that I only told my closest friends about (most gastrointestinal and urinary, I deemed these embarrassing and inappropriate for public consumption). In fact, I didn't even write about these side effects explicitly in my private documents, choosing instead to hint at them as a way of keeping a record that they existed. For instance, I wrote the following in a private Word document dated January 20, 2020, the day I completed chemotherapy:

My best friend says it's like "insult to injury" that this sort of thing happens – like it's not bad enough to have cancer but then this shit happens on top of it. But I'm not injured (even though I realize the injury here is metaphorical); I do have an illness, and it is not metaphorical. I begin to adapt and use her phrase constantly, almost daily, "insult to illness" – as each day I endure some sort of harm, small or large, that seems either absurd or almost unbearable, and always some addition to the shit-show of what I'm already dealing with – having cancer, going through chemo – as if it can't get worse, there's always some additional insult.

Here, I attempt to resist metaphors in my writing as a way to empower myself against illness. Susan Sontag (1978) claims, in *Illness as Metaphor*, "the metaphors attached to… cancer imply living processes of a particularly resonant and horrid kind" (p. 9). The body becomes a host for a tumor, a growth, undergoing "a process in which the body was consumed" (p. 10). An opaque (p. 12), de-sexualized, degenerating (p. 13), body subject to mutilation, amputation, and death (p. 15). Sontag wants us to resist metaphors, and thus I do, writing, "I do have an illness, and it's not metaphorical," connoting instead that it is real unlike the metaphorical "injury," which can be emotional or physical, in the commonplace, "insult to injury." In changing the phrase to "insult to illness," meaning not just something bad happening on top of a vague something bad, but something bad happening on top of a specific thing—cancer—I attempt to assert some power over the side effects that come with cancer treatment.

Co-mingling with the reflection stage of the process here, my writing does not necessarily indicate acceptance. One doesn't need to accept themselves as ill in order to understand that their body is ill. In that same sentence about metaphor, my writing demonstrates a need to ground my illness in material reality, yet I do not say, "I am ill." The use of "I have" versus "I am" is an important epistemological distinction, denoting that an illness is separate from the person—something they can have and then eventually not have—and not something that defines them, something they are. This is similar to the above example, where I refer to "the cancer" instead of "my cancer"—it's a way of understanding cancer as separate from oneself.

Reflection

At the time I'm writing this (February 2023), it has been almost exactly three years since I completed chemotherapy and radiation treatments, and again I am considered "cured." In that time, the world has suffered from the COVID-19 pandemic. As a recently treated cancer patient with a highly at-risk immune system in Spring 2020, I spent the first many months of the pandemic terrified that if I got the virus, it would kill me. As time has gone on, I'm less scared, but I nonetheless suffer from the long-term physical and emotional effects of "surviving" breast cancer. As I wrote recently in *Rhetoric of Health & Medicine*:

> Often thankful to be alive, grateful for "no evidence of disease" (NED), now labeled a "survivor," patients still suffer. Now we suffer not from the treatment, but from the chronicity of the treatment, the "demoralizing change from a person who has an illness to someone who is an illness" (Estroff, 1995, cited in Smith-Morris, 2010, p. 25). The chronicity of chemo means every cell in our being has been pricked; and we are now essentially transformed.
>
> (Siegel Finer, 2022, p. 162)

That transformation comes not only from having gone through the treatment but from having gone through the epistemological process of being ill.

Here, I attempted to craft a rhetorical autoethnography that offers ways to understand and acknowledge how a patient comes to understand her identity as a patient, which happened to me through the patient epistemology cycle. Somewhat surprisingly, my experiences neatly map onto the cycle of patient epistemologies we describe throughout this book, and having gone through that process has helped me tremendously. It helped me grapple with questions like: how do I come to understand what's going on in my body, what's being done to me by my medical team, and how I'm being treated by my friends and loved ones? How do I make meaning from this, and/or make this meaningful? Am I different now? This is also where we see rhetorical autoethnography as an apt example of how time, space, and effort (in writing in this case) can feature in the meaning-making process. Writing this chapter has helped me to see that writing throughout my cancer experience was an epistemological experience, mostly because it helped me cope with the absurdity of a lot of the cancer experience, how cancer can consume a life in unpredictable ways and in ways that are aporetic because of cancer's demands.

Woolf (1926) writes:

> Considering how common illness is, how tremendous the spiritual change that it brings, how astonishing, when the lights of health go down, the undiscovered countries that are then disclosed, what wastes and deserts of the soul a slight attack of influenza brings to light, what precipices and lawns sprinkled with bright flowers a little rise of temperature reveals, what ancient and obdurate oaks are uprooted in us in the act of sickness, how we go down into the pit of death and feel the waters of annihilation close above our heads and wake thinking to find ourselves in the presence of the angels.
>
> (p. 32)

Woolf does not take illness lightly, using intense words and phrases like "astonishing," "pit of death," and "annihilation" to describe illness. Yet, coming out of illness is so revered, it is as if being "in the presence of the angels" (p. 32). I argue that this "waking" she refers to does not happen by itself. We wade in the "waters of annihilation," meaning that waking happens through our suggested process of patient epistemologies, where one experiences a health flashpoint, does rhetorical work to understand their identity as a person with an illness, grapples with material and constitutive effects, and then reflects on their new reality, new health status (not necessarily improved), new understandings of themselves and loved ones, etc. So, while being sick is perhaps transformational in itself, I believe that the research and writing I did while ill is what helped, perhaps, to have a more nuanced understanding of my experience even while "down into the pit of death."

I hope the take-away from this autoethnography is that writing while sick is a valuable part of being sick; accepting the flashpoints framework is helpful in accepting illness. Woolf (1926) says that "they [ill people] would complain that there was no love in it—wrongly however, for illness often takes on the disguise of love" (p. 33). She claims that it's too scary to look illness in the face, that one "would need the courage of a lion tamer," and that it's scary to take time to write about illness as it's not lovely or romantic (p. 33). However, I have found that doing so is transformational, or as Woolf says, "this monster, the body, this miracle, its pain, will soon make us taper into mysticism, or rise, with rapid beats of the wings, into the raptures of transcendentalism" (p. 33). It is less so that Woolf's metaphors speak to us, but rather her consideration of one's self, one's emotions, one's reality and sense of reality; her urge and maybe even need to make meaning of illness through rhetorical efforts— all things we have argued need imbuing into RHM and care-givers' attention to women's health experiences to better support them.

References

Childs, P., & Fowler, R. (Eds.). (2006). *The Routledge dictionary of literary terms.* Routledge.

Ehrenreich, B. (2009). *Bright-sided: How positive thinking is undermining America.* Metropolitan Books.

Hensley Owens, K. (2019). Writing my body, writing my health: A rhetorical autoethnography. In J. White-Farnham, B. Siegel Finer, & C. Molloy (Eds.), *Women's health advocacy: Rhetorical ingenuity for the 21st century* (pp. 14–24). Routledge.

Lunceford, B. (2015). Rhetorical autoethnography. *Journal of Contemporary Rhetoric, 5*(1/2), 1–20. http://contemporaryrhetoric.com/wp-content/uploads/2017/01/Lunceford10_1.pdf

Murray, S. J. (2009). Aporia: Towards an ethic of critique. *Aporia: The Nursing Journal, 1*(1), 8–14. https://www.researchgate.net/publication/26645036_Aporia_Towards_an_Ethic_of_Critique

Pender, K. (2018). *Being at genetic risk: Toward a rhetoric of care.* The Pennsylvania State University Press.

Segal, J. Z. (2008). Breast cancer narratives as public rhetoric: Genre itself and the maintenance of ignorance. *Linguistics and the Human Sciences*, 3(1), 3–23. https://doi.org/10.1558/lhs.v3i1.3

Siegel Finer, B. (2016). The rhetoric of previving: Blogging the breast cancer gene. *Rhetoric Review*, 35(2), 176–188. https://doi.org/10.1080/07350198.2016.1142855

Siegel Finer, B. (2018, January 12). Five years after breast cancer, a survivor feels cut off from the care that kept her safe. *The Philadelphia Inquirer*. https://www.inquirer.com/philly/health/five-years-after-breast-cancer-a-survivor-feels-cut-off-from-the-care-that-kept-her-safe-20180111.html?query=bryna%20siegel%20finer

Siegel Finer, B. (2019, December 26). Sabbatical side project. Blogging BRCA: The BRCA experience in real time. https://bloggingbrca.wordpress.com/2019/12/

Siegel Finer, B. (2019, June 29). For my next trick. Blogging BRCA: The BRCA experience in real time. https://bloggingbrca.wordpress.com/2019/06/29/for-my-next-trick/

Siegel Finer, B. (2019, July 11). Missed my calling. Blogging BRCA: The BRCA experience in real time. https://bloggingbrca.wordpress.com/2019/07/11/missed-my-calling/

Siegel Finer, B. (2019, July 2). Life (and death) goes on. Blogging BRCA: The BRCA experience in real time. https://bloggingbrca.wordpress.com/2019/07/02/life-and-death-goes-on/

Siegel Finer, B. (2020, Nov 6). (Not) Choices. Blogging BRCA: The BRCA experience in real time. https://bloggingbrca.wordpress.com/2020/11/06/not-choices/

Siegel Finer, B. (2022). "I've never felt right after chemo": The chronicity of post-chemotherapy. *Rhetoric of Health & Medicine*, 5(2), 161–180. https://www.muse.jhu.edu/article/859971

Smith-Morris, C. (2010). The chronicity of life, the acuteness of diagnosis. In L. Manderson & C. Smith-Morris (Eds.), *Chronic conditions, fluid states: Chronicity and the anthropology of illness.* (pp. 21–38). Rutgers University Press.

Sontag, S. (1978). *Illness as metaphor*. Farrar, Straus and Giroux.

Woolf, V. (1926). *On being ill*. The New Criterion.

Afterword
Looking to the future of patient epistemology

Biographical life and biological life, as we argue in the second chapter of this book, are too often conceived of as separate and separable, and this cleaving makes health flashpoints particularly fraught. That is, when a health flashpoint enters the scene with all of its attendant affect, the stories we tell ourselves about our lives—where we are going, what our future looks like, who we are—and the way we live in these physical bodies each day slam into each other in ways that can feel violent. As we have also noted, the pace of contemporary life, swathed in neoliberal leanings, too often encourages people to ignore or delay attention to our bodies and to push forward with life no matter the circumstances. Indeed, many signs around us suggest that our worth is directly tied to remaining productive in the capitalist sense regardless of circumstances. Yet, our human bodies don't always allow that kind of efficiency, and hyper-productivity hardly promotes wellness. Disability scholars describe this conundrum eloquently and theorize "crip time" as an alternative orientation to the chronological; crip time has a relationship to the cycle of patient epistemologies in that our theory is similarly attempting to trace temporal intricacies that are difficult to articulate. Crip time signals "the complexity of disabled experience in a world with many barriers to accessibility" (LeRoy, 2021).

Some writers have described the way crip time can present as "moments out of time, out of productive, forward-leaning, exciting time" (Kuppers, 2014, p. 29). Others make it clear that crip time can be liberatory, but it can also feel like loss and alienation (Samuels, 2017). Margaret Price (2021) has relatedly discussed the concept of what she calls "accommodation loops" wherein individual accommodations alongside biomedically-driven surveillance allow for the possibility that the ableism in workplaces is never addressed. That is, if a person's time is taken up with seeking accommodations at an individual level, and the person is also subjected to invasive questions about why they require accommodations in the first place, less attention goes to making institutions less ableist. Such circumstances necessitate crip time, a space to operate outside of what are considered "normal" temporalities. Crip time calls attention to the ways that temporality and affect intertwine and complicate each other; as a theoretical construct, it does so in a way that highlights the damaging and

DOI: 10.4324/9781003398318-7

ableist assumptions about what human beings are and what their lives are for. Crip time and related theories also allow for more generative and inventive ways of engaging in the temporal. As J. Logan Smilges (2023) put it,

> My thinking on time and feeling is informed by conversations in disability studies and Mad studies on how people's experiences of disability, trauma, and madness can contour their relationships to temporality … Taken together, crip time, trauma time, and mad time capture the affectivity of temporality, the dimension of feeling with/in time and sensing time with/in feeling.
>
> (p. 25)

In the same way, the cycle of patient epistemologies as we have described it allows for a different orientation to patients and how they navigate health flashpoints differently than traditional studies of patient education materials have. A new diagnosis, a worsening of an existing condition, or the progression of a natural process can make ableist notions of temporality and forward movement feel impossible and absurd. Lingering and deliberating on information, likewise, has benefits. As this book has argued, health flashpoints that give way to cycles of patient epistemologies often overlap and entangle with others as few of us are fortunate enough to face one at a time. For those with one or more chronic health conditions or disabilities, of course, the cycle is long, ongoing, and incredibly knotty. In the affect-laden rhetorical work that must be performed, there needs to be space to explore crucial sources of information and forms of support that might lead patients to make the best decisions for themselves, for those they care for, and for their communities. When discourses and affect collide in real time, and when life keeps pushing forward at a punishing pace, it can be difficult, in that context, for patients to find, consider, and use the information and support that is needed to make such decisions.

As an example, Cathryn has had uterine fibroids for decades, and they cause a wide variety of issues that are burdensome, but they are also considered benign as they aren't deadly or actively causing harm to body systems. Symptoms include extreme bloating, feelings of fullness with abdominal distension, heavy bleeding, and cramping. As those who've also suffered from especially large fibroids know well, clinicians often compare fibroids to various fruits when describing their relative size to their patients. While myomectomies (or surgical procedures to remove fibroids) can be performed, such procedures are not without risk, and fibroids inevitably grow back—at least until menopause—and continue to wreak havoc in a variety of ways. One of Cathryn's fibroids, considered a "grapefruit," was removed through such a surgical intervention in 2014, yet many more grew back in its place. Even though she, at that time, had no plans for another child, doctors strongly pushed for the uterine sparing options, such as hormone-blocking medications and myomectomy—instead of a hysterectomy due to her age. As rhetoricians of health and medicine have noted, women of childbearing age are often strongly discouraged from any interventions that might harm fertility—even when they tell their care providers that they don't want any (or any more) children, and especially in instances in which they are seeking elective sterilization without having had any children (Davis & Dubisar, 2019).

The worsening of an existing condition—uterine fibroids—constituted a health flashpoint that necessitated information and support, and in the affectively overwhelming space of sorting out options, Cathryn opted for the myomectomy even though she might have pushed for a hysterectomy if that had been presented as a legitimate option. Co-occurring depression along with the stress of the first years on the tenure track made considering other options feel impossibly consuming. Removing the large fibroid, moreover, changed her fertility in ways that she did not fully comprehend and was complicated by the fact that hormonal birth control makes her incredibly ill. Therefore, in 2017, Cathryn experienced an unplanned pregnancy that was, as many people pointed out at the time, a "total game changer" in terms of her and her family's plans for the future. At 37 and with a nearly 16-year-old son, this pregnancy brought with it a wave of hormones that led to even more fibroid growth along with the dreaded pregnancy condition known as "hyperemesis gravidarum," or persistent and severe vomiting that leads to repeated dehydration, drastic weight loss, and hospitalizations.

Overwhelmed with the pregnancy for a variety of reasons and trying to prepare a tenure dossier made the frequent ultrasounds to monitor the fibroids growth vis-à-vis the fetus growth into passing curiosities rather than occasions for real thought on treatment options, and no mention of treatment options were ever made. We are always at the mercy of what information and support exist as we are thrust into discourse communities that are not of our own choosing. Now, six years later, the fibroids are more intrusive than ever, and Cathryn's providers are suggesting a full hysterectomy. Yet this treatment should have been offered as an option initially in 2014, and, more importantly, while the pregnancy progressed, perhaps care providers might have suggested a c-section with hysterectomy right then and there rather than wait until the fibroids became unbearable. Future choices about surgery will be complicated by the care of Cathryn's now five-year-old, similar to what our breast cancer patients recalled.

When affect and information collide at the same time that a person's plans for their life have been completely altered and they must continue to pay bills, do their jobs, and care for their children, pets, parents, and communities, it is crucial that they have all of their options presented to them in a clear way and that the supportive systems around them function to make good rhetorical work and deliberation possible. Doing otherwise can cause continued suffering in ways that are also present in the people we were fortunate enough to speak with in our focus groups, such as our participant who was never presented with flat closure as an option post-mastectomy and ended up later regretting her breast reconstruction. While it may seem like, in both cases, the women should have thought of and advocated for the best option on their own, the cycle of patient epistemologies uncovers the complexities inherent in such rhetorical work, making it all too clear how much better support persons need to do with considering how they themselves contribute and perhaps critique sources of information and forms of support in health. As the menopause discourses we examined make clear, intrusive and repeated messaging in *doxa* can foreclose on the possibility of more and better information or, indeed, progress. In the case of Cathryn's fibroids situation (which is ongoing), the *doxa* that says that women of childbearing ages should not be offered hysterectomies, but perimenopausal women should be pushed toward them, makes a difference in how cycles of patient epistemologies deploy.

Tracked through a variety of health conditions and realities, this book has helped to better articulate those sources of information and forms of support that help patients through the overwhelming rhetorical work that goes along with health flashpoints. Some of us do experience long phases of life that are unremarkable in terms of health. As we (the authors) navigate our 40s, we are aware of times in our own lives in which health flashpoints felt fewer and further between. Yet no one fully escapes health flashpoints, and some, such as those with ongoing disabilities and/or chronic conditions, are overburdened with them and their attendant capacity to alter affective, cognitive, and physical lives forever—particularly because the imperatives in place for how we ought to live our lives are so very ableist.

As the women in our breast cancer focus groups make clear, far from the linear narrative arc from diagnosis to wellness, their experiences of/with breast cancer treatments have forever altered them. Menopause, too, constitutes a life-altering transition; substance use disorder also creates a wide variety of changes in and for the individual sufferer. Thinking of these health flashpoints as constitutive pieces of human life that involve affect-laden rhetorical work and cyclical, frenetic activity helps us to better articulate the sources of information and forms of support that could be most advantageous. However, in crafting our theory of patient epistemologies, we have been mindful of the limits of "awareness." We are not merely attempting to point out what might help versus what might hurt when a person faces a health flashpoint, be it a health crisis in the form of a dire diagnosis, the worsening or flare of an existing and/or chronic health condition, or the progression of a natural process that presents new symptoms. Instead, we are theorizing that what happens in these moments is significant as there is a disruption in day-to-day life that draws attention to the precarity of human existence that contradicts the pace of contemporary life. Biographical life is cleaved from biological life. A person's life as they've known or imagined it has shifted, and identities have altered.

This book has been an attempt to provide a theory of how critical health decision-making unfolds rhetorically—from the time of a health flashpoint through to reflection. It is our hope that the theory we have provided will be an accessible research tool for future study in a variety of health and medical contexts and beyond. Moreover, while the conditions this book takes up as cases through which to theorize a cycle of patient epistemologies are mostly discussed as they unfold for an individual sufferer, we see broader implications and applications for this theory in public health framings. For example, we might consider the COVID-19 pandemic as something of a global health flashpoint such that we can better track how discourses, affect, and information collided with everyday life as it was rapidly changing.

Likewise, as we write the conclusion to this book during the summer of 2023, the world is contending with the promises and perils of Artificial Intelligence (AI) and its potential impacts on all areas of life, including patient education and patient-provider communication. Indeed, some are making the provocative suggestion that AI may have better "bedside manner" than human care providers (Devlin, 2023). In thinking through what role AI might play in patient care, education, and critical decision-making, the cycle of patient epistemologies offers a useful framework for future study. That said, global pandemics and AI are only two small examples of the broad applications to which the theories developed in this book might contribute. As we continue our own inquiries into the conditions that help or hurt rhetorical and identity work in the context of health flashpoints, for instance, we are increasingly attracted to the idea of utilizing the theory of patient epistemologies to study the role that stigma—a longtime area of interest for RHM scholars—plays in health and help-seeking behaviors (Cole & Carmon, 2019; Cook et al., 2021; Kessler, 2022; Miller, 2019; Molloy, 2019; Walkup & Cannon, 2018). We hope that other writers in health communication, rhetoric of health and medicine, health humanities, and related fields use the theory as a generative framework in the same way.

References

Cole, K. L., & Carmon, A. F. (2019). Changing the face of the opioid epidemic: A generic rhetorical analysis of addiction obituaries. *Rhetoric of Health & Medicine*, 2(3). https://doi.org/10.5744/rhm.2019.1014

Cook, C., Scott, B., Holic, N., Sukhija, M., & Woody, A. (2021). Evaluating the use of comic storyboards to create educational materials about stigma for health care providers. *American Public Health Association 2021 Annual Meeting and Expo*.

Davis, S., & Dubisar, A. M. (2019). Communicating elective sterilization: A feminist perspective. *Rhetoric of Health & Medicine*, 2(1). https://doi.org/10.5744/rhm.2019.1004

Devlin, H. (2023, April 28). AI has better 'bedside manner' than some doctors, study finds. *The Guardian*. https://www.theguardian.com/technology/2023/apr/28/ai-has-better-bedside-manner-than-some-doctors-study-finds

Kessler, M. M. (2022). *Stigma stories: Rhetoric, lived experience, and chronic illness.* The Ohio State University Press.

Kuppers, P. (2014). Crip time. *Tikkun, 29*(4), 29–30. https://doi.org/10.1215/08879982-2810062

LeRoy, T. (2021, November 30). *What is Crip time?* Accessibility.com. https://www.accessibility.com/blog/what-is-crip-time

Miller, E. (2019). Too fat to be president? Chris Christie and fat stigma as rhetorical disability. *Rhetoric of Health & Medicine, 2*(1), 60–87. https://doi.org/10.5744/rhm.2019.1003

Molloy, C. (2019). *Rhetorical ethos in health and medicine: Patient credibility, stigma, and misdiagnosis.* Routledge.

Price, M. (2021). Time harms: Disabled faculty navigating the accommodations loop. *South Atlantic Quarterly, 120*(2), 257–277. https://doi.org/10.1215/00382876-8915966

Samuels, E. (2017). Six ways of looking at crip time. *Disability Studies Quarterly, 37*(3). https://doi.org/10.18061/dsq.v37i3.5824

Smilges, J. L. (2023). *Crip negativity.* University of Minnesota Press.

Walkup, K. L., & Cannon, P. (2018). Health ecologies in addiction treatment: Rhetoric of health and medicine and conceptualizing care. *Technical Communication Quarterly, 27*(1), 108–120. https://doi.org/10.1080/10572252.2018.1401352

Index

Page numbers in **bold** denote tables, those in *italic* denote figures.

110   *Index*

Taylor & Francis Group
an **informa** business

Taylor & Francis eBooks

www.taylorfrancis.com

A single destination for eBooks from Taylor & Francis
with increased functionality and an improved user
experience to meet the needs of our customers.

90,000+ eBooks of award-winning academic content in
Humanities, Social Science, Science, Technology, Engineering,
and Medical written by a global network of editors and authors.

TAYLOR & FRANCIS EBOOKS OFFERS:

A streamlined
experience for
our library
customers

A single point
of discovery
for all of our
eBook content

Improved
search and
discovery of
content at both
book and
chapter level

REQUEST A FREE TRIAL
support@taylorfrancis.com

Routledge
Taylor & Francis Group

CRC Press
Taylor & Francis Group

For Product Safety Concerns and Information please contact our EU
representative GPSR@taylorandfrancis.com
Taylor & Francis Verlag GmbH, Kaufingerstraße 24, 80331 München, Germany

www.ingramcontent.com/pod-product-compliance
Lightning Source LLC
Chambersburg PA
CBHW061828220326
41599CB00027B/5223

*9 7 8 1 0 3 2 5 0 3 9 6 7 *